Mucuna versus Parkinson:

Treatment with Natural Levodopa

Dr. Rafael González Maldonado

2

MUCUNA versus PARKINSON:

Treatment with Natural Levodopa

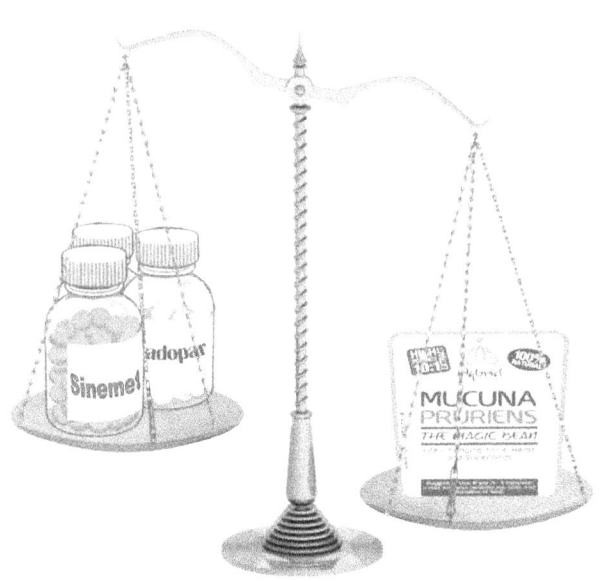

Dr. Rafael González Maldonado

TITLE: *Mucuna versus Parkinson. Treatment with natural levodopa*

AUTHOR: **Rafael González Maldonado**

Cover design: Julio González Valverde

Illustrations: Claudia González Durán

Photo: Carlos González Durán

Edited: Amazon (CreateSpace)

Buy online: www.amazon.com , www.amazon.es

1st EDITION: August 19, 2014.

ISNB 10: 1500938114
ISBN 13: 9781500938116

©*Copyright 2014*: Rafael González Maldonado.
All rights reserved. rafael@gonzalezmaldonado.com

Images: personal & variations from CreativeCommon and Pixabay.com

---

WARNING: DISCLAIMER: *The below uses are based on tradition, scientific theories, or limited research. They often have not been thoroughly tested in humans, and safety and effectiveness have not always been proven. Some of these conditions are potentially serious, and should be evaluated by a qualified healthcare provider. There may be other proposed uses that are not listed below. The concepts and data in this book are not optional suggestions or recommendations but subject to errors or guesses debatable, and must be contrasted with the judgment of the physician. This information is not specific medical advice and just try to help clarify health concerns; are based on review of scientific research data, historical practice patterns, and clinical experience should not be followed by a patient or acquaintance without consulting the responsible physician must consider each individual case, with the history, medications and patient's clinical situation and monitor inconsistencies or errors in dose.*

Creeds and schools in abeyance,
retiring back a while sufficed at what they are,
but never forgotten.

SONG OF MYSELF (Walt Whitman, 1892)

◆ ◆ ◆

Me aparto de las escuelas y de las sectas,
las dejo atrás; me sirvieron, no las olvido.

CANTO DE MÍ MISMO (Traducción de J.L. Borges)

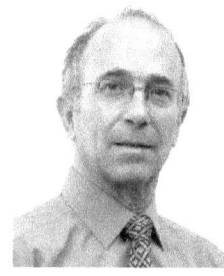 Dr. Rafael Gonzalez Maldonado is a neurologist with an extensive professional career: Doctor of Medicine, Honorary researcher at the Royal Free Hospital (London), Professor of Medicine, Chief of Neurology at the University Hospital of Granada (1991-2005). He currently is a neurologist at private practice.

He has written several popular books of Parkinson's disease: "The strange case of Dr. Parkinson", "Unorthodox Treatments for Parkinson's Disease" "Parkinson and Stress," "Conjectures of a Neurologist who Listened a Thousand Parkinsonian patients" as well as numerous scientific publications.

He has also edited bilingual texts with translation into Spanish of the classic English and French: "An essay on the shaking palsy" (Parkinson 1817), "*De la paralysie agitante*" (Charcot and Vulpian, 1862) and "*De la maladie de Parkinson*" (Denombré, 1880).

"*Mucuna versus Parkinson: Natural Levodopa Treatment*" is so far the most complete and up-to-date monograph on the subject, it describes the theoretical and practical approaches to the use of this plant as a treatment option for Parkinson's disease. Also included are more than one hundred of references.

Index

Introduction

1. A brief history of levodopa
2. Beans contain levodopa
3. Mucuna, a bean that grows in the tropics
4. From the herbalist's shop to the pharmacy
5. Mucuna works better than Sinemet
6. Extracts of mucuna patented by neurologists
7. Contraindications and warnings
8. Dosage and presentations
9. Testimonials from those who take Mucuna
10. How to start taking Mucuna: cases studies
11. The future of Mucuna
12. Buy Mucuna *online*. Do consultations

Bibliography
Table of contents

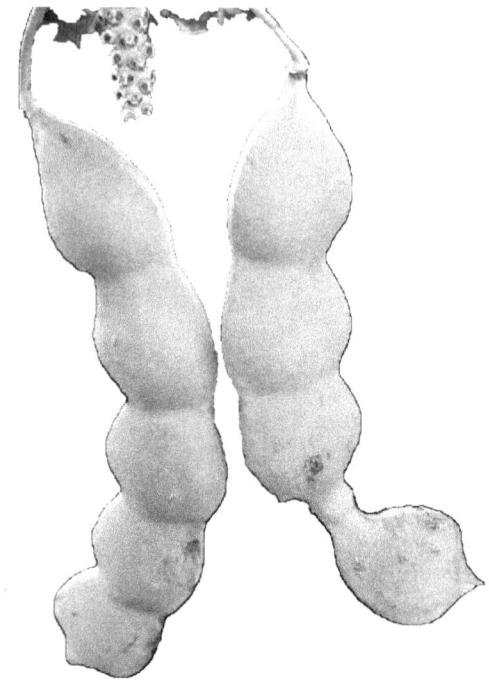

Mucuna is a bean (Leguminosae) that grows in the tropics and contains levodopa naturally in large quantities. Mucuna improve symptoms in many people with Parkinson's disease.

Introduction

Mucuna is a species of bean that grows in the tropics. It is very rich in natural levodopa, which is better tolerated and more potent than the synthetic levodopa in Sinemet, Madopar or Stalevo.

Mucuna seeds extract has been an effective treatment of Parkinson's disease in many patients. The fact that its use is not widespread is due not only to ignorance of the part of the patients and lack of communication from physicians, but also because the pharmaceutical industry has shown no interest yet for various reasons. However, one can expect its application to spread in coming years. Scientific studies attest to it and renowned neurologists such as Dr. Warren Olanow and Dr. Andrew Lees have patented, in Germany and the United States, the specific techniques for extracting levodopa from this plant.

Meanwhile, patients have recorded their positive experiences with mucuna; they buy it online (no prescription needed) and use it in secrecy without consulting their neurologist. Neither the patients nor the doctors (most of them) have clear ideas about this plant, its ingredients (not only levodopa), the proportions in which it is absorbed, or how to manage it.

Mucuna is used without control, and if there are not more accidents is because it is relatively safe (although there are risks if misused), and most of the capsules sold contain very low doses, almost like a diet supplement. The formula at high concentrations is dangerous, especially when mixed with antiparkinsonian drugs. Be careful what you buy, where you buy it, and what the dosage is. Do not combine drugs without medical advice.

Mucuna is not just an herbal product of Ayurvedic medicine. Allusions made here to hindu medicine are mainly historical. Currently, extracts from the seeds or leaves are not strange alternative therapies but rather an important part of the treatment of Parkinson's disease, and they hold great promise for the coming years.

The above mentioned patent *"relates to the use of Mucuna pruriens seeds for the preparation of a pharmaceutical composition for the treatment of Parkinson's Disease to obtain a broader therapeutic window in L-Dopa therapy, to delay a need for combination therapy, to obtain an earlier onset and longer duration of L-Dopa efficacy, and to prevent or alleviate acute and chronic L-Dopa toxicity"*.

The full description of this patent (WO 2004039385 A2) and references that support it can be found at:

http://patentscope.wipo.int/search/en/WO2004039385

If you or someone you know has Parkinson's you need to know about mucuna, its important advantages and few disadvantages and, above all, you must know how to use it to benefit many (not all) patients with Parkinson's disease.

That is the purpose of this book.

Rafael González Maldonado.

Granada, August 19, 2014.

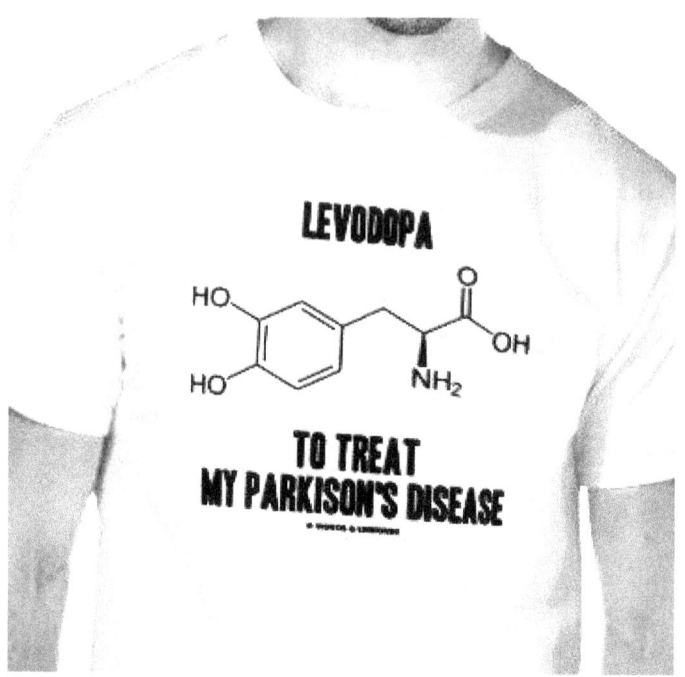

LEVODOPA IS THE BEST TREATMENT

Levodopa is a natural substance contained in meat and some plants, which use it to defend themselves. Discovered by Guggenheim in beans in 1913, it remains the best treatment for Parkinson's disease.

1. A brief history of levodopa

Dr. Guggenheim felt sick. He noticed that his pulse was racing and he had to vomit. He thought, and rightly so, that it was because he had eaten too many beans.

He had the idea of analyzing them in his laboratory and then learned that he had discovered a new amino acid, dihydroxy-phenylalanine or levodopa [1]. It was unevenly deposited in the plant, the pods containing more than seeds. This happened in 1913.

LEVODOPA IS CONVERTED TO DOPAMINE

From the biological point of view levodopa was apparently inactive. A growing interest in 1938 followed the discovery of an enzyme, decarboxylase, which turns levodopa into dopamine, the first active amine in the chain of catecholamines.

PARKINSON'S PATIENTS LACK OF DOPAMINE

Hornykiewicz, from whom I copy the title of this chapter [2] made several findings around 1960: the brain of

Parkinson's patients, particularly the basal ganglia, contains greatly decreased amounts of dopamine [3], which is a neurotransmitter essential for motor coordination.

DOPAMINE INCREASED AFTER TAKING LEVODOPA

The next step, after an initial hesitation, was to try oral administration of levodopa. It was found that dopamine ascended to the brain and that people with Parkinson's disease improved dramatically: the shaking stopped and their walking improved miraculously. But there was a serious problem, their nausea and discomfort were hardly endurable.

BEGINNING TO WALK, THEY BEGAN TO VOMIT

I was a child when my father, a great doctor in a small village (beautiful Almuñécar), so proud of his profession, showed me Larodopa, the medication given him by a delegate from Roche Laboratories.

"*This makes walking some who are paralyzed by Parkinson's disease, although it provoked vomiting and they feel very bad.*"

Larodopa contained only synthetic levodopa. After crossing through the duodenum to the blood, levodopa reaches the brain, and allows the parkinsonian to walk. However, it also reaches the intestine, heart and other organs, causing vomiting, tachycardia, and an overall sorry state.

That memory never faded and I found a miracle when I saw people paralyzed for years who, when beginning to walk, began to vomit.

SINEMET AND MADOPAR PREVENT VOMITING

Dopamine (not levodopa) improves the symptoms of Parkinson's disease. We need to increase dopamine in the brain since it improves the rigidity and tremor, but it it is preferable that the dopamine not remain in the blood or the rest of the body because it can cause vomiting, tachycardia, and other uncomfortable symptoms.

To prevent vomiting and other ailments Sinemet (from Latin *sine* and *emetere* words: without vomits) came to the fore. The trick was to add another substance to the levodopa, carbidopa, which inhibits decarboxylase (it destroys the destroyer) and prevents levodopa from being converted to dopamine.

As carbidopa does not cross the blood-brain barrier, it does not affect brain dopamine, but it inhibits the formation of dopamine in the blood. That way the brain receives the benefits of dopamine and other organs do not suffer damage.

PATIENTS TREATED WITH SYNTHETIC LEVODOPA

Levodopa remains the most powerful drug with synergistic dopaminergic effects [4]. I am going to describe the drugs containing levodopa in the summary, although I admit that reading this synthesis is boring.

To this end, I write in small print, in an attempt to alert the reader that these paragraphs are expendable and can be skipped, but it can be consulted by anyone with enough curiosity and patience.

FOUR TYPES OF SINEMET

Sinemet is the best-known parkinsonian mediation. The different proportions of levodopa and carbidopa (inhibitor of decarboxylase which prevents its conversion to dopamine) should take into account.

Sinemet 25/250 was the original presentation and the name means that there are 25 milligrams of carbidopa (inhibitor) for every 250 mg of levodopa (a dopamine precursor substance); the proportions are 1:10.

As some patients continued to have nausea with this combination, the ratio was changed to 1:4, the so called Sinemet Plus 25/100:

carbidopa 25 mg to 100 mg of levodopa. It produces less nausea and other side effects and is preferable for beginning the treatment.

There are also two forms S.R. (which slowly release their contents into the intestine): Sinemet Plus Retard 25/100 and Sinemet Retard 50/200. In both cases the ratio 1:4 was chosen (greater proportion of inhibitor, fewer side effects).

LEVODOPA + BENSERAZIDE (MADOPAR)

This is the preferred formula of France and other European countries. The system is the same: the adverse effects of dopamine are decreased here by benserazide, a substance having an action very similar to the carbidopa.

The commercial product is called Madopar 50/200, i.e. each tablet has 50 mg of the inhibitor (benserazide) and 200 milligrams of levodopa. It is therefore a high proportion of inhibitor (1:4), similar to Sinemet Plus. The same ratio is used in the delayed release form: Madopar Retard 25/100.

"STABILIZED" LEVODOPA (STALEVO)

This is another system used to maintain stable levels of levodopa. If Sinemet Retard slows absorption from the intestine into the blood, Stalevo decreases the elimination of plasma levodopa by the liver and kidneys. This is accomplished by adding entacapone to levodopa and carbidopa.

The entacapone, which initially was used separately (Comtan 200 mg) inhibits catechol-amino-transferase that promotes metabolism (the elimination) of levodopa. As the disposer is removed, levodopa remains in the blood for a longer period of time, and the improvement of patients lasts for several hours.

Its predecessor was tolcapone (Tasmar), a very effective drug that is not already distributed in many countries because of its serious side effects. Entacapone gives an orange color to the urine that has no negative effect. Commercial success came when these substances were combined in the same tablet: Stalevo "100" for example, is a mixture of a Sinemet Plus (100 mg of levodopa and 25 mg carbidopa) with 200 mg of entacapone.

Stalevo 50, 100, 125, 150, 200, 225, etc. are the names of different doses of levodopa. These doses provided the proper proportion of carbidopa, but every tablet contain 200 mg of entacapone.

Stalevo is theoretically the most efficient way of administer levodopa. It was supposed that as it prevent fluctuations in plasma levels of levodopa, it would decrease subsequent occurrence of dyskinesias; this is something that other studies put in doubt,

LEVODOPA AS A DEFENSE AGAINST ITS NEIGHBORS

Levodopa is not abundant in nature. Why are some plants generating levodopa? To defend themselves and to attack other vegetables. Levodopa is a precursor to many alkaloids, catecholamines and melanin, and when the plants produce levodopa they use it to eliminate other plants that compete with them in the same terrain [5].

Levodopa from some legumes (such as beans) destroys the roots and shoots of the neighboring plants [6] that are growing in the field and also to repel insects [7]. It is a weapon of defense and attack between plants to mark their territory, is a system for setting limits otherwise known as allelopathy [8] [9].

OTHER PLANTS CONTAINING LEVODOPA

Common beans have sufficient amount of levodopa to produce significant clinical effects but, as we will see, *Mucuna pruriens* (and other varieties) have a very high content of levodopa.

Levodopa is also found in many species of plants, although in much lower concentration: *Vigna aconitifolia, Vigna unguiculata, Vigna vexillata, Prosopis chilensis, Pileostigma malabarica, Phanera vahlis, Parkinsonia acculeata, Mucuna urens, Canvavalia glandiata, Cassia floribanda, Casia hirsute, Dalbergia retusa,* etc. [10]

Research on their efficacy remains to be done in animal models.

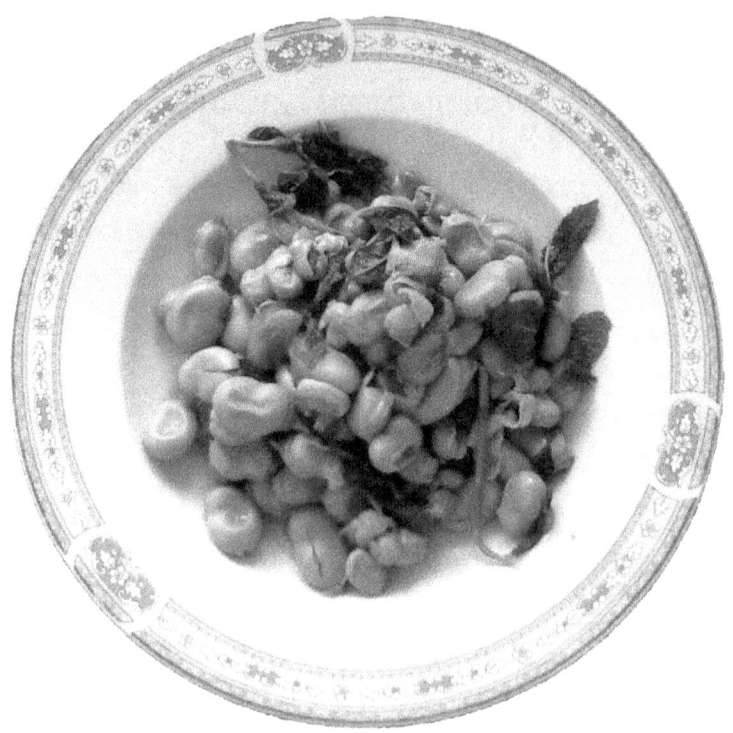

A SERVING OF BEANS EQUIVALENT TO HALF A TABLET OF SINEMET

Common beans contain levodopa in its seeds and pods, but in low concentrations. This proportion is much higher in the buds. A serving of beans may accumulate as much levodopa as half a tablet of levodopa Sinemet.

2. Beans contain levodopa

Gugenheim ate beans with natural levodopa. Later, the pharmaceutical industry manufactured synthetic levodopa that is sold as Sinemet, Madopar and Stalevo.

Common beans (*Vicia faba*) are a natural source of levodopa, which accumulates in the pods and in the seeds, although in apparently small amounts.

CONSUMING BEANS IMPROVES PARKINSON'S

There was anecdotal descriptions of Parkinson's patients who experiences improvements after consuming beans [11].

The first controlled trial demonstrating efficacy was carried out in 1992. The researchers asked several Parkinson's patients to eat a serving of beans, and then measured blood levodopa. They found that, parallel to the rise in blood levels of levodopa, symptoms improved at the same time [12].

A SERVING OF BEANS IS HALF A SINEMET

This is the equivalence in terms of the improvement of symptoms and of the elevation in blood levels of levodopa.

In one study [12], six Parkinson's patients (at a median of 63.5 years old, 13 years of duration of disease, all at stage 3) were left without medications for 12 hours. Then they ate a dish of cooked beans (half a pound).

In the next four hours there was an increasing level of levodopa in the blood while the symptoms improved. This amelioration was similar to that which took place a few days later, under the same conditions, but giving half of a tablet of Sinemet 25/250 mg, i.e, 125 mg of levodopa with carbidopa 12.5 mg.

It is believed that in early-stage Parkinson's disease, with few symptoms, beans would be a choice of treatment [13]... if you find a way of ingesting the necessary quantities.

JUST A LITTLE LEVODOPA WORKS

Common beans contain low concentrations of levodopa that theoretically would disappear rapidly from the blood because the decarboxylase enzyme immediately converts it into dopamine.

It is therefore strange what we have seen: a small amount of levodopa that is ingested by eating beans suffices to improve parkinsonian symptoms. The simplest explanation is that these patients also take Sinemet, which contains carbidopa, and this substance increases the effectiveness of the levodopa in the vegetable.

But, why does this also occur in patients taking only agonists of dopamine without Sinemet? I will explain below.

LEVODOPA PLUS CARBIDOPA IS MORE EFECTIVE

In addition to levodopa, beans contain some carbidopa [14] (which reduces decarboxylase enzyme). Therefore levodopa can remain in the blood longer before becoming dopamine.

That explains the improvement experienced by the patients: it is because beans contain levodopa and carbidopa in combination (more so in the tender sprouts).

In a way, the beans mimic Sinemet but perfect it. Within their seeds the carbidopa / levodopa ratio is 1:1. In Sinemet that ratio is 1:10, and in Sinemet Plus is 1:4. Taking into account these proportions, beans resemble a "super-plus" Sinemet.

It is recommended that the daily dose of carbidopa contain between 75 and 200 mg for fear that their clinical effects would be reduced due to excessive inhibition of dopa-decarboxylase.

However, recent studies show that the parkinsonian symptoms continue to improve under a daily dose of 450 mg carbidopa [15]. This would be a way to decrease the peripheral side effects of levodopa. In some countries tablets containing only carbidopa (Lodosyn) are dispensed. It has also been found that the absorption of carbidopa varies among individuals. Some people assimilate in "fast" mode and others in "slow". This may explain variations in the response [16] between individuals and the daily clinical oscillations observed. This could perhaps be corrected with an additional dose of carbidopa.

BEANS ENRICHED WITH CARBIDOPA

It is a good idea. We have seen that beans contain a naturally beneficial levodopa but in a limited quantity. This means that a little levodopa may improve symptoms because it has combined with the high proportion of carbidopa (it inhibits the decarboxylase that clear levodopa from the blood). It was recommended, always under medical supervision, that the patient eat some sprouts combined with carbidopa to increase efficiency: thus they needed fewer beans and parkinsonian symptoms improved more [14].

Good research on this has been done in Australia [17]. They have enriched beans with synthetic carbidopa and the results are much more evident: six patients ate a serving of beans mixed with carbidopa and five of them, in 40 minutes, marked an improvement of motor control which lasted almost two hours, equivalent to that which occurred when they were given one tablet of Sinemet.

In addition, plasma levodopa levels increased in parallel with the ingestion of carbidopa tablet [17] and beans.

POWDERED DRY BEANS HAVE LITTLE LEVODOPA

The attempt to treat parkinsonian symptoms with levodopa from common beans raises two problems.

The first is common sense: if a quarter of a kilo (about nine ounces) of beans is equivalent to half of a Sinemet 25/250, the average patient ought to take in between one and two kilograms (i.e. between two and four pounds) of beans daily.

The other option is to dry the legumes to be pulverized later. This does not work because dry beans contains less levodopa, and then they cannot be compressed into capsules. The patient would have to take it in bags, many bags, and that is not practical.

SEEDBED TO COLLECT BEAN SPROUTS

The young beans contain more levodopa than the mature ones but there is even much more in new sprouts of seedlings.

If seeds are prepared for germination and bean sprouts are collected, the extract obtained is quite rich in levodopa [18], almost 20 times more.

With these it is found that plasma levels rise demonstrably and symptoms improve. The maximum level of levodopa is achieved on the sixth day after soaking the seeds in water [19]. There is another great advantage: buds are digested better than seeds and uncomfortable flatulence avoided.

Some patients grow their own beans in private gardens, but can be accomplished with a large seedlings. Bean seeds germinate quickly and easily, and every morning one may harvest a dozen emerging sprouts: a small treasure to take as a daily dietary supplement.

Varieties of beans are also tested to increase their content of levodopa [20]. It is an economical choice that has already been **proposed** [101] for developing countries where Sinemet, Madopar or Stalevo are too expensive.

DOSAGE MUST BE ADAPTED TO EACH CASE

Many patients can benefit from the consumption of beans, under medical supervision, taking into account the contraindications (favism or other previous illnesses, incompatible drugs, etc.). Also we must understand that the dosage is highly variable as it will depend on many factors.

The amount of levodopa can vary greatly by species, area of cultivation, soil conditions, precipitation and other factors. Is known that young bean pods contain more levodopa than mature grain. Approximately 100 g (3½ oz) fresh or green beans, may contain 50 to 100 mg levodopa [18].

BEANS ARE MORE EFFECTIVE IN PATIENTS

Even if the beans are tender, with more levodopa, a healthy person hardly notice it. Its effect, however, is much higher in Parkinson's patients medicated with Sinemet, Madopar or Stalevo (these tablets, bearing carbidopa, increase the effectiveness of levodopa beans, as we have seen).

Researchers have described some cases in which a patient with levodopa and dopamine agonists, after consuming the tender beans that they collected, were hospitalized with symptoms of severe dyskinesias [21].

Eating beans changes the clinical state of the patients, sometimes too. And, if taken under controlled conditions, it can improve daily motor fluctuations.

NEUROLEPTIC SYNDROME AFTER CESSATION OF BEANS

Eating beans influences the functional state of people with Parkinson's disease, as we have seen in the previous case of overdose. But there is also evidence of the opposite case: a parkinsonian had been taking beans as adjuvant therapy for months, and suddenly interrupted the consumption. That caused a neuroleptic malignant syndrome (fever, rigors, lethargy, etc.), [22] the same clinical picture that occurs when a patient stops taking their medication abruptly.

BEANS REDUCE "ON-OFF" FLUCTUATIONS

We have seen that in some patients who take various drugs (levodopa, dopamine agonists and others) eating broad beans can produce uncontrolled dyskinesias, because of the interactions that occur.

As published in the respected journal Movement Disorders, it has been shown that, under supervision, moderate consumption of beans decreases the clinical fluctuations of patients, prolonging the "on" time, i.e. the period of time they feel better [23].

Typically, 100 grams (four ounces) of fresh beans a day is sufficient [24], but if you choose this option to improve your Parkinson's disease, and especially if you use extracts, you must do so gradually and always under medical supervision since it may be necessary to adjust previously prescribed medications. Eating beans without medical advice carries risks [25], including overdose, allergies and others.

SEARCHING FOR PLANTS WITH MORE LEVODOPA

The ideal would be to find plants (legumes or others) with a higher content of levodopa. This solution exists but not in European countries: in India, tropical Africa, and the Caribbean a wild legume grows, a "hairy bean" which has ten times more levodopa than ours: *Mucuna pruriens*. We shall see it in the next chapter.

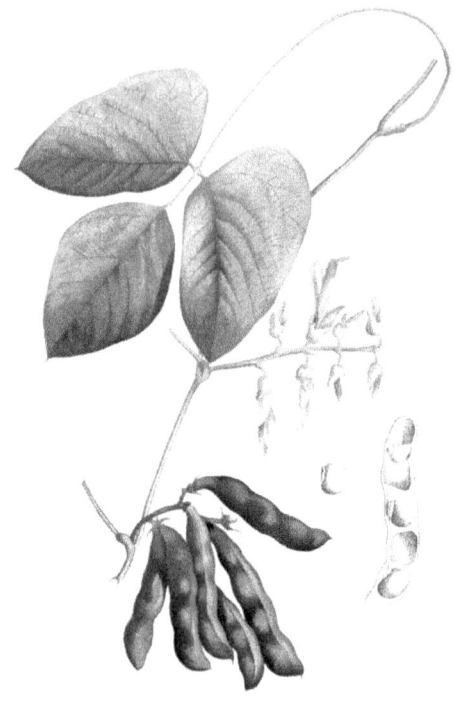

MUCUNA, A BEAN THAT GROWS IN THE TROPICS

It is a legume, a "hairy" bean, with pods covered by fuzzy fibers that cause intense itching if they contact the skin ("*pruriens*"). It contains lots of natural levodopa and it is a choice to treat some people with Parkinson's disease

3. Mucuna, a bean that grows in the tropics

Levodopa, a direct precursor of dopamine, is the main medication for Parkinson's disease. Patients are treated with "synthetic" levodopa in different doses or combinations in tablets of Sinemet, Madopar and Stalevo.

The largest natural source of levodopa is Mucuna, a legume (such as common beans, peas, lentils, peanuts). Extracts from the variety of *Mucuna pruriens*, especially the seeds, display a very interesting biochemical profile. These have been used for three thousand years in more than 200 recipes from India medicine.

Extract of mucuna seed powder contains large amounts of levodopa and a little serotonin and nicotine along with other ingredients that are only partially known. In the treatment of Parkinson's disease such extracts seem to be more effective and less toxic than the synthetic preparations [26].

FURRY BEAN GROWING IN THE TROPICS

Mucuna pruriens is a kind of "hairy" or furry bean, native to Southeast Asia, especially the plains of India, but also widely distributed in tropical regions of Africa and the Americas (particularly in the Caribbean).

The wide dissemination of the plant explains its variety of names, depending on the location: velvet beans, cowhage, itch bean, picapica, Fogareté, Kapikachu, sea bean, deer eyes, yerepe, Atmagupta, nescafe, chiporazo.

A SHRUB AS A VINE

This annual plant grows as a climbing shrub with long tendrils that enable it to reach more than fifteen feet in height.

Young plants are almost completely covered by a diffuse orange hair that disappears as they age. It grows or is cultivated as fodder to enrich the soil (adding a lot of nitrogen) or for its medicinal qualities.

Since its discovery [27], in 1937, and due to its high content of levodopa, interest has grown and now it is produced in much larger quantities.

ITS FLOWERS ARE POLLINATED BY BATS

The velvet bean leaves are of the trifoliate type, with leaflets of 5 to 12 cm (4 in.) in width and 7-15 cm (3-5 ") long.

The white or purple flowers are in axillary racemes up to 32 cm long. They are self-fertile, though in some places they are pollinated by bats which, while trying to eat nectar of the plant, carry pollen from flower to flower in their ears [28].

PODS AND SEEDS

The pods are produced in groups of 10 to 14, measure 4-13 cm long and 1-2 cm wide, and are covered with fine white or light brown hairs.

Each capsule contains 3 to 7 seeds, which are from 8 to 13 mm wide and 10 to 19 mm long [29]. The seeds can be black, white, red, brown or mottled.

NAMED "PRURIENS" BECAUSE OF THE ITCH

It is called "pruriens" because of the intense itching produced by their contact.

The orange "hairs" of flowers and pods of *Mucuna pruriens* contain chemicals (including serotonin) that, when they come in contact with the skin, cause intense irritation and itching, and sometimes very troublesome injury including allergies and severe swelling.

FOOD, FORAGE OR GREEN MANURE

Velvet bean or mucuna is mainly used as a cover crop or green manure, which provide organic matter and nitrogen to the soil. Fresh biomass yields are high.

Mucuna pruriens produces nematicidal compounds and can reduce the population of worms when combined with other crops. This also has allelopathic effects that suppress weed growth.

Another use of mucuna is as a high quality forage. In fields where the pods are mature sheep and goats can graze.

Its leaves, pods and seeds are high in protein, much more so than any of the other pasture grasses. Interestingly, if the proportion of mucuna is high the animals reach a slightly lower weight [30] [31] suggesting some toxic or disnutritive element.

The roasted seeds are used as a substitute for coffee in areas of Central America. The buds and young pods are used as food after being cooked several times.

The dried seeds can be consumed after being soaked in water for 24-48 hours and then cooked [29], changing the water several times to reduce the content of toxic and antinutritive compounds.

AN ANCIENT MEDICINE

In India, mucuna has been the main healing herb for three thousand years. All parts of the plant are used in more than 200 indigenous medicinal preparations. The seeds contain up to 7% levodopa, which is used in the treatment of Parkinson's disease.

In the Ayurvedic medicine, velvet bean is recommended as an aphrodisiac, and studies have shown that its use causes a rise in testosterone levels, increased muscle mass and strength, and also improves coordination and attention.

TOXICITY OF MUCUNA AND OTHERS LEGUMES

The difference between a drug and a poison is a matter of dosage. The appropriate dose of levodopa improves Parkinson's and other diseases, but when taken in excess it may cause problems.

Ingestion of large amounts of vegetables (of the *Fabaceae* type) by any person may induce intoxication because an excess of levodopa, when converted into dopamine, provokes abdominal symptoms (pain, vomiting) and cardiovascular abnormalities (tachycardia, flushing, etc.). These symptoms have been described in common beans and also in different varieties of mucuna, e.g. *Mucuna gigantea* [32], originally from Hawaii.

LEVODOPA AND MORE

The interest in mucuna increased after 1937 when it was discovered [27] that the variant contained large amounts of levodopa. However, this amino acid alone does not justify the many medical applications of this interesting plant.

Extracts from the seeds or other parts of the plant have many numerous healing properties that cannot be explained only by levodopa.

In the treatment of Parkinson's disease some results in groups of patients and in experimental animals show that, apart from natural levodopa, *Mucuna pruriens* has other ingredients that show outstanding features. It must contain other substances that improve the absorption of levodopa and metabolic efficiency, as explained below.

50 KNOWN INGREDIENTS, OTHERS REMAIN

Mucuna pruriens is an amazing plant. In addition to levodopa, it contains other natural ingredients that influence their particular properties, although some are found in small quantities.

To date, 50 substances have been identified in the powder of its seeds [33] [34] [35] [36]. Other still unidentified components must exist in mucuna, such as portions or mixtures of alkaloids, proteins, peptides, polysaccharides, glycosides, glycoproteins and several phytochemicals including tryptamine, alanine, arginine, glutathione, isoquinolone, mucunine, nicotine. prurienine, serotonin, tyrosine, etc. [37]

These substances, identified or not, confer special powers on mucuna, perhaps boosting the levodopa or adding some kind of dopamine agonism and even extended its effects. We need to continue investigating them.

OTHER PLANTS THAT CONTAIN LEVODOPA

It was thought that levodopa was only present in Mucuna (*Vicia* species), but it can also be found, although less concentrated, in plants like *Phanera, Cassia, Pileostigma, Canavalia, Dalbergia,* etc.[38] This extends the horizon for new therapies.

However the differences among these are striking. It has been well known for a long time that beans contain natural levodopa, although in small quantities, and may improve some parkinsonian symptoms. Our beans, when they are green, including pod and seeds, contain 0.6% concentration of levodopa.

The whole fruit of *Mucuna pruriens*, contains a concentration of 4.02 %, and if you select the white variant of its seed, it contains 6.08 % levodopa (ten times higher than in common beans) [38].

MUCUNA CONTAINS MORE LEVODOPA

Trials have been conducted in which mucuna seeds are germinated in darkness or in different conditions of light and providing varied nutrients (oregano, proteins from fish, etc.).

Results showed that by adding oregano to seeds germinated in darkness, mucuna sprouts containing 33% more levodopa have been obtained [39].

In an attempt to increase the proportion of levodopa in mucuna, researchers selected some cells from the ground, and then grew them grow in a medium that allow nutrients to be supplied.

In this way they have managed successfully to increase the concentration [40] [41] [42].

MUCUNA CAN PROVIDE OTHER BENEFITS

This is a question of common sense. If, apart from levodopa, *Mucuna pruriens* naturally contains certain substances that make it more effective, the same can happen with other varieties of mucuna (there are many) or with other vegetables that have been capable of modifying the proportions of levodopa, antioxidants and other ingredients [43] [44].

This opens up a horizon of new therapeutic possibilities.

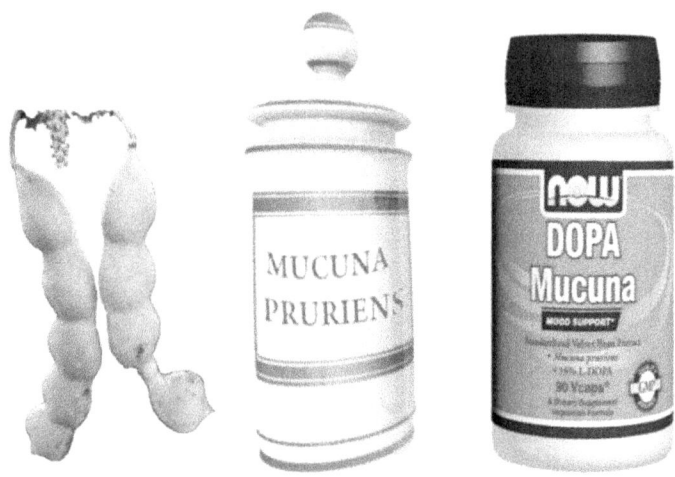

FROM THE HERBALIST'S SHOP TO THE PHARMACY

Mucuna would no longer be considered just an herbal supplement but a good drug to be dispensed at pharmacy. It contains natural levodopa having many advantages over the synthetic.

4. From the herbalist shop to the pharmacy

This is not a book of Hindu medicine so, with a blatantly practical approach, I'll strip the mucuna, this amazing herb, from everything that reminds one of Ayurveda.

I respect this ancient health system but, in this book, I wish only to tap into the experience accumulated over the centuries during which many people have been treated with mucuna extracts. These contain useful substances for Western medicine, in particular for the treatment of Parkinson's disease.

Ayus (r) means life and *veda* is knowledge. Ayurveda is "knowledge of life". It is a holistic system about man, health, and longevity that was developed in India three or four thousand years ago.

This Hindu health system considers the body as a whole in which disease is caused by intrinsic or external harmful elements. Therapy is based on special diets and practices, especially the application of a variety of herbs and very interesting drugs.

HERBS THAT HEAL

The Hindus used a root extract of *Rauwolfia serpentina* to lower blood pressure and as a tranquilizer.

Without discussing the theories of Ayurveda, laboratories CIBA (Basel, Switzerland) analyzed the plant and acquired reserpine, a drug that was a milestone and that launched a revolution in the treatment of arterial hypertension [45] [46].

That is what we intend to do with mucuna, a forest vine, actually a legume, which contains, naturally, levodopa, the main treatment for Parkinson's disease.

We will study the experience of current practice in the use of mucuna, and we will try to take advantage of the potential benefit for people with Parkinson's disease.

Thousands. or hundreds of thousands, of patients treated with mucuna for centuries are evidence that the side effects of these seeds are not frequent or severe.

MUCUNA AS PANACEA

Panacea, the daughter of the physician-god Asclepius, had accompanied him with a sort of kit bearing different remedies for all diseases. This is similar to features attributed to mucuna, which is recommended in Ayurveda to treat more than 200 diseases: as a vital tonic, an aphrodisiac, a remedy to reduce stress, a good diuretic... and is also used against parasites, to control diabetes and lower cholesterol. And, of course, it is a treatment for *kampavata* (the equivalent of Parkinson's disease).

Western science seems to confirm many of these effects. Mucuna improves libido, semen quality... and even works against snake bites.

GROWTH HORMONE BOOSTER

Mucuna increases the adaptation and regeneration of tissues in general, and has been shown to increase growth hormone [47].

It has an anabolic effect and increases muscle mass; it also has antioxidant properties and favors the protective functions of the liver [48].

LOWERING OF CHOLESTEROL AND GLUCOSE.

Diabetics and people with high cholesterol may benefit from mucuna [49]. In rats has been shown to lower cholesterol by 61% and glucose was reduced by 39% [50][51].

Mucuna enhances the recovery of diabetic neuropathy induced in animals [52]. In humans it delays the onset of diabetic nephropathy. Mucuna also protects the stomach to relieve gastric mucosal lesions induced experimentally in rats [53].

AN APHRODISIAC THAT IMPROVES SEMEN

Mucuna increases libido, or sexual drive, in men and women due to its dopamine-inducing properties; dopamine is the substance of desire and profoundly influences all appetites.

In male animals Mucuna raises testosterone levels and increases sexual activity [54] [55] [56].

In men with fertility problems mucuna clearly enhances sexual drive and power while improving the quality of the sperm: it increases the number of cells and also gives them greater mobility [57] [58]. It is assumed that it act on the hypothalamus-pituitary-gonadal axis.

IT ACTS AGAINST EPILEPSY AND AGAINST CATALEPSY

Researchers can cause status epilepticus or catalepsy in experimental animals by various techniques: electroshock, pilocarpine or Haloperidol). These improve if treated with velvet beans [59].

SNAKE POISON ANTIDOTE

This is not an exaggeration or a myth. Mucuna is a good antidote for snake bites, possibly by a direct effect on the venom, attributed to its glycoprotein antitrypsin content [60] but also because it is procoagulant and prevents cardio-respiratory depression induced by poison.

Specifically, Mucuna reduces mortality due bites from the following snakes: Gariba viper (*Echis carinatus*) [61], Viper Malaya [62] and spitting cobra (*Naja sputatrix*) [62] [63] [64].

IMPROVES BOWEL MOVEMENT

Mucuna contains prurienine which increases intestinal peristalsis and is a good remedy for constipation, so prevalent in Parkinson's patients.

It usually enhances motility and gastric emptying, although some patients assert otherwise.

KAMPAVATA IS PARKINSON'S DISEASE

In India there were Parkinson's patients three thousand years before the birth of James Parkinson. These were diagnosed as *Kampavata*, a disease characterized by trembling (*Kampa* in Sanskrit). In Ayurveda this process was classified within the group of neurological disorders (*Vata Rogas*) [65] [66].

They obviously lacked Sinemet and Madopar but were treated naturally with levodopa, obtained by crushing mucuna seeds, which they later diluted and administered as a beverage [65] [67]. For thousands of years this therapy has worked, these patients have improved and, above all, according to that we know, showed fewer side effects than people taking synthetic drugs.

ITS NAME WAS ATMAGUPTA

It has become popular to call the plant "mucuna". This word is of Guarani origin (after the name of a vine in the Amazon) but in India the original denomination of this plant is *Atmagupta* or *Kapicachhu*, and it is still sold on some websites under this name.

Different extracts of its seeds were used against tremor or rigidity; and also as an aphrodisiac or an antidote to the venom of the cobra or other snakes.

There are other herbs that Hindus used to treat different symptoms of Parkinson's disease such as constipation, insomnia, anxiety and others: *Plantago psyllium, Ulmus fulva, Glycyrrhiza glabra, Withania somnifera,* etc.

AYURVEDA IN TREATING PARKINSON

As we said, we will not delve into Hindu medicine, but some general aspects of Ayurveda may be useful in Parkinson's patients.

For this disease, along with herbal remedies, full therapy requires a change of lifestyle and daily regimen in order to be in harmony with one's personal constitution. The true intention is that the patient achieve a physical and mental balance, and this in some way helps cure the disease

THE SEEDS ARE COOKED IN COW'S MILK

In an interesting clinical trial, 18 Parkinson's patients were treated according to the criteria of Ayurvedic medicine.

They received a concoction of powder of *Mucuna pruriens* cooked in cow's milk along with other traditional plants (*Hyoscyamus reticulatus, Withania somnifera, Sida cordifolia*) [68].

The results found that this treatment improved rigidity and bradykinesia, tremor was diminished and cramps subsided; however sialorrhea (drooling or excessive salivation) worsened.

Later, the powder of plants which had been added to the milk was analyzed and it was found that each dose used contains 200 mg of levodopa [68].

HIDDEN INGREDIENTS IN MUCUNA

The Hindu mucuna extract contains a small amount of levodopa that fails to justify the significant clinical improvement of parkinsonian symptoms.

This suggests that in the mucuna there are other substances that enhance the role of levodopa (such as carbidopa, entacapone or tolcapone) or other active ingredients with antiparkinsonian effects [67] [69] [70].

This is the same as we have discussed regarding common beans. In them, the amount of levodopa is too low but it is effective because the legume has other substances that enhance its effects; it is also possible the beans are associated with some ingredients that inhibit the enzymes that metabolize the levodopa, maximizing its effectiveness.

Similarly, and possibly to a greater extent, we see the effect of the *Mucuna pruriens* itself: apart from natural levodopa, it has other substances that, one way or another, improve the parkinsonian symptoms and reduce side effects [69].

In another chapter we will study some of the substances that accompany levodopa in mucuna, although there are others that are not yet known.

One important thing is guaranteed by Ayurveda: after thousands of years of using these plant extracts, thousands or millions of patients have continued to improve their symptoms without significant adverse effects.

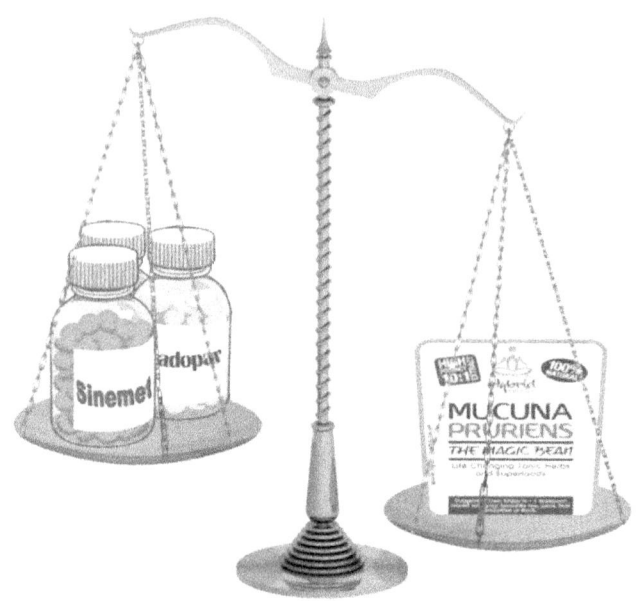

MUCUNA WORKS BETTER THAN SINEMET

In rats it has already been shown. In people there is much evidence about the advantages of mucuna as has been found in well-designed and scientifically based trials.

5. Mucuna works better than Sinemet

There is growing evidence in support of mucuna extracts as a natural medicine for the treatment of Parkinson's disease.

FIRST DESCRIPTIONS

In 1978, a publication by R.A. Vaidya in India stated that Parkinson's disease could be treated with extracts of a plant, *Mucuna pruriens*, which contains natural levodopa and is tolerated better than the synthetic version [71].

In the West the scientific writings that described improvement in parkinsonian symptoms after eating mucuna or other beans appear between 1990 and 1994 and are authored by B.V. Manyam, J.M. Rabey and P.A. Kempster [13] [17] [65].

In the first edition (January 1997) of one of my popular medical books, *The Strange Case of Dr. Parkinson* [72], I have previously commented on these findings.

In the chapter implicatively entitled *Beans instead of pills*, I emphasized that these legumes could replace some of the conventional medication. I have also included some recipes from "Parkinsonian Cuisine" that are based on beans. In some of my other books, I have references to further publications on the subject [69].

MUCUNA SEED POWDER

Scientific journals have begun publishing cases of improvement in patients after eating mucuna. The Parkinson's Disease Study Group undertook a multi-center clinical study (in collaboration with several hospitals) with 60 patients, of which 26 took Sinemet before the test and the other 34 were "pharmacologically virgins" (they had never taken levodopa).

All were treated for 12 weeks with powder from mucuna seeds: an average of 6 bags, each containing 7.5 grams, equivalent to 250 mg of levodopa. In other words, each sachet contained the same amount of levodopa as a Sinemet 25/250, but without the carbidopa.

Neurologists of four centers screened patients using the appropriate scales (UPDRS) and found considerable improvement that was statistically confirmed. [73] Thus,

Ayurveda medicinal recipes have demonstrated their clinical effectiveness.

ZANDOPA: A MEDICINE WITH MUCUNA

This legume seems to work. Investigations gave evidence of this and mucuna seed powder (called HP-200) was marketed as a drug, under the brand name Zandopa. [34]

It was first distributed in India, and has been available in the United Kingdom since 2008. Now customers can buy it freely online without a prescription. It is important to be careful, however, because the levodopa dose is relatively high (250 mg per sachet) when combined with carbidopa or other antiparkinsonian drugs (see the description of Zandopa below).

IMPROVEMENT IN MICE DOUBLES OR TRIPLES

We can experimentally induce parkinsonism (unilateral or bilateral) in rodents via certain toxic substances. Used in these trials, levodopa from mucuna has no side effects and produces an improvement that is double or triple that of the synthetic version. [74]

This also suggests that mucuna can contain components that enhance the action of levodopa (as when combined with carbidopa, entacapone or tolcapone). There is another possibility: namely that mucuna itself, regardless of its levodopa content, relieves the parkinsonian symptoms.

In another experiment, animals ate extract of mucuna for a year. They were then put down and their neurotransmitters were measured in different areas of their brains.

Interestingly, no changes were seen in the nigrostriatal pathway, but dopamine was significantly increased in the cerebral cortex. [34] This has two possible explanations: that natural levodopa is more potent, or that mucuna contains other beneficial chemicals.

ENDORSED BY THE AMERICAN ACADEMY

This clinical study [26] complies with the strict requirements laid down by the most rigorous scientific methodology established by the Quality Committee of the American Academy of Neurology [75].

This was a randomized, double-blind, crossover, study which adhered to precise objectives and clearly defined protocols, and was carried out by several independent observers.

They studied 8 Parkinson's patients at (on average) 62 years of age, 12 years after diagnosis with a stage of progression of 3.5 on the Hoehn & Yahr scale. Prior to this test they were treated with levodopa (572 mg mean value). In addition, patients were taking others previous associated drugs (amantadine, pergolide, ropinirole, pramipexole or cabergoline) that remain unchanged. All had a rapid response to levodopa (1.5 to 4 hours) along with very disabling motor fluctuations during the morning.

Each subject was hospitalized three times (one week apart) and went without any medication the night before the test. The next morning, at the same time, each received at random one of three combinations: one dose of 200 mg of levodopa with 50 mg of carbidopa (two tablets of Sinemet Plus), or two or four sachets of mucuna (15 or 30 grams) equivalent to 500 or 1000 mg of natural levodopa (100 or 200 according to the conversion factors).

The results were clearly better in those who take two sachets of mucuna extract: improvement in their symptoms occurred faster, their plasma levodopa levels were higher, and clinical efficacy was more durable. In addition, their dyskinesia was not worsened. The details follow.

"CITIUS, ALTIUS, FORTIUS ET DURABILIUS"

The Olympic motto *"faster, higher, stronger"* can be applied to mucuna, because, in comparison to Sinemet, it acts more rapidly (34 minutes instead of 68), produces a greater elevation of the plasma level of levodopa (110% higher), and appears to be stronger (the effectiveness of natural levodopa is double or triple that of the synthetic version).

In addition, the improvement achieved is more durable (with mucuna the "on" phase is prolonged 37 minutes longer than with Sinemet). Therefore, it can be described as *Citius, altius, fortius... durabilius*.

TWICE AS EFFECTIVE

We have seen that the mucuna seed extract naturally contains levodopa. If we quantify and compare it to the same dose of synthetic levodopa contained in tablets of Sinemet (or Madopar) we find that levodopa from mucuna is approximately twice as powerful in controlling parkinsonian symptoms. [10]

The efficacy of synthetic levodopa (without carbidopa) has been compared to that of natural levodopa (mucuna) using rats with experimentally induced parkinsonism. The natural levodopa proved to be two times as effective at improving symptoms [76]. This test maintained the following proportions: 125 and 250 milligrams of synthetic levodopa were compared with the equivalent dose of natural levodopa (respectively, 2.5 and 5 grams of mucuna powder 5%).

This means that in addition to levodopa, mucuna provides other substances (with carbidopa-like or other properties) that increase its effectiveness.

Then the test was repeated, this time adding 50 mg of carbidopa to the two types of levodopa. Again, mucuna proved to be more efficient.

THE PROBLEM OF VOLUME

Mucuna is more effective, more rapid and durable, however... to achieve a dose that will offer the same relief as Sinemet or Madopar, it would be necessary to prescribe large amounts of seed powder dissolved in liquid [71] [77]. The need to consume seed powder several times a day would soon overwhelm the patient and the treatment would be abandoned as too cumbersome.

The solution to the problem can be found in concentrated extracts. This allows for the presentation of mucuna in tablets or capsules, facilitating the application of different doses of the product and making it easy to manage daily consumption of mucuna in the amounts deemed necessary.

There is another choice that requires the cooperation of the neurologist: mucuna could be used in association with carbidopa to achieve greater efficiency with less seed powder.

We will see more on this further ahead.

MUCUNA WITH CARBIDOPA

The first trials that compared the effects of Sinemet with mucuna required six or seven daily sachets of powdered seeds. This can be maintained for a few days, but becomes quite cumbersome with time.

Actually those studies were done to compare natural levodopa (mucuna) to a synthetic combination of levodopa and carbidopa (i.e. the contents of Sinemet).

The solution seems simple: add carbidopa to mucuna. This increases the efficiency of the natural levodopa contained therein and therefore eliminates the need to take large amounts of seed powder.

We must be careful when capsules of concentrated extracts are used because the dose can be excessive when you consider that mucuna is more effective than synthetic levodopa [26].

There are published trials in which mucuna is administered in combination with carbidopa and is compared to Sinemet.

Rats with experimentally induced hemi-parkinsonism were treated with powdered mucuna seeds (2.5 and 5 g) associated with carbidopa (50 mg) and in contrast to other groups wherein the equivalent synthetic levodopa dose (125 and 250 mg) was also associated with carbidopa.

Mucuna-carbidopa proved to be more than twice as effective as Sinemet and this was found by measuring the rotation contralateral (on the injured side) of the animals in each group [76].

We know that the carbidopa in Sinemet prevents the peripheral side effects of levodopa (nausea, rapid heart rate) and enhances mobility. It appears that, the carbidopa in mucuna is even more effective: it decreases mild side effects and doubles or triples patients' strength [26].

MUCUNA DOES NOT PRODUCE DYSKINESIA

A different study, this time in monkeys (with unilateral parkinsonism induced experimentally), produced very interesting results on the possibility of dyskinesias.

One group was treated with Sinemet (levodopa and carbidopa), another with mucuna plus carbidopa, and the third only with mucuna. All the animals experienced an improvement in their symptoms.

Dyskinesia was then assessed by the study of spontaneous activity in the substantia nigra. Larger dyskinesia appeared in the Sinemet group. In those treated with the combination of mucuna and carbidopa dyskinesia seemed more moderate. Interestingly, in those who had only taken mucuna no dyskinesia was found. [33]

LONG-TERM MUCUNA WITHOUT DYSKINESIA

A similar experiment was performed, but this time mucuna treatment was continuous, extending for a year. It was done in rodents and compared mucuna with Madopar.

One group was treated with Madopar (levodopa and benserazide), another with mucuna plus benserazide, and the third only with mucuna.

All were controlled for a year. The symptoms were alleviated in all groups, but the improvement was significantly higher in those who were treated with mucuna plus benserazide.

To highlight the results of long-term use: after one year, major dyskinesia appeared in rats that had taken Madopar. Rodents treated with mucuna plus benserazide had some minor dyskinesia. Animals that took only mucuna ... none at all [78].

This suggests that the mucuna contains unknown ingredients that produce effects similar to those of benserazide (or carbidopa), or which, for some reason, reduce the need for this association in order to improve parkinsonian symptoms.

MUCUNA IMPROVES HALOPERIDOL-INDUCED DYSKINESIA

As previously mentioned, mucuna extracts do not produce dyskinesia after long-term treatment, but it seems that there is another advantage.

In an experiment with different dyskinesia (those produced by neuroleptics like haloperidol) these repetitive movements improved when mucuna was administered [79].

MUCUNA IS NEUROPROTECTIVE

Most clinicians believe that levodopa (the synthetic version thus far used) is harmful due to a possible association with increased free radical formation.

Some authorized opinions disagree and express doubts about the myth of "toxic levodopa" in cases where low doses are used.

Well, it seems that natural levodopa from mucuna (or the whole of the components in this legume) is non-toxic, and even neuroprotective [80].

This has been demonstrated in mice (with experimentally induced parkinsonism) which were given synthetic levodopa or mucuna.

Those treated with mucuna experienced an improvement in most of the symptoms. Also, when they were slaughtered one year later for brain analysis it was found that the endogenous contents of levodopa, dopamine, norepinephrine, and serotonin in the *substantia nigra* was significantly restored [35].

These results have been attributed to other ingredients in mucuna known to protect against Parkinson's disease: NADH (nicotinamide adenine dinucleotide) and coenzyme Q-10.

CHELATING AND ANTIOXIDANT PROPERTIES

In other studies with rodents, researchers agree that the extract of mucuna clearly is neuroprotective compared to synthetic levodopa [81] or estrogen [82].

They believe that this is due to its antioxidant and chelating activity (processing of iron), and because it avoids mutagenic effects in DNA [83] [84].

MUCUNA IMPROVES BRAIN FUNCTION IN RATS

Antioxidant and neuroprotective properties of mucuna has also been shown in rodents that were previously damaged experimentally by nerve toxins such as Paraquat.

The results also highlighted the improvement in habits and cognitive functions of these animals [85].

DOSAGE DOES NOT INCREASE OVER TIME!

It sounds too good to be true: treatment with mucuna does not produce dyskinesia; and it also improves secondary abnormal movements which occur with chronic synthetic levodopa therapy.

One more thing: with mucuna it would be not necessary to gradually increase the dose as time goes on, as is the case with those taking synthetic drugs.

Below, I transcribe literally the benefits of mucuna extracts as reflected in the scientific foundations of the patent carried out by Van der Giessen, Olanow, Lees and Wagner [37]: we are going to discuss this more broadly in the following chapter:

"Conventional L-Dopa therapy requires a gradual increase of the effective dose over time resulting of progression of disease and/or the neurotoxic effects of L-Dopa or dopamine with an increase of toxic reactions and, over time, the appearance of dyskinesia, increasing in severity with dose. In clinical experiences with Mucuna prurience seed preparations these negative phenomena have not been observed in that for the effective treatment of Parkinson's, the dose of Mucuna pruriens derived L-Dopa remained relatively stable over longer periods of time, and in that dyskinesia, even in patients with pre-existing dyskinesia

following long term therapy with conventional L-Dopa preparations, appeared to be less in occurrence and severity..." [37]

After reading this, it seems strange that mucuna is not yet dispensed in all pharmacies as a revolutionary drug.

Patentes francés inglés

Mucuna pruriens and extracts thereof for the treatment of neurological diseases
WO 2004039385 A2

Número de publicación	WO2004039385 A2
Tipo de publicación	Solicitud
Número de solicitud	PCT/EP2003/010975
Fecha de publicación	13 May 2004
Fecha de presentación	2 Oct 2003
Fecha de prioridad	30 Oct 2002
También publicado como	CA2504201A1, 6 más »
Inventores	Andrew Lees, Waren C Olanow, Der Giessen Rob Van, Hildebert Wagner

---

EXTRACTS OF MUCUNA HAVE BEEN PATENTED

Two renowned neurologists and a professor of Phytomedicine have patented a mucuna seed extract to treat Parkinson's disease.

6. Extracts of mucuna patented by neurologists

Thousands or millions of Parkinson's patients have been treated with mucuna for millennia in Hindu medicine. From what we know, the results have been good and with few side effects.

That experience has drawn the attention of several neurologists since 1990, and launched serious clinical studies which have subsequently confirmed the benefits of Indian herbs.

Experiments with rats have also shown that natural levodopa improved symptoms and produced less neurological damage than the synthetic version. It was concluded that extracts of *Mucuna pruriens* contain high concentrations of levodopa and it are more effective and better tolerated with fewer side effects.

My conversion to the expectations of mucuna became definitive when I discovered that two very famous neurologists (Dr. C. Warren Olanow and Dr. Andrew Lees) had patented these extracts in Germany and the

United States. These physicians are recognized worldwide as the foremost experts on Parkinson's disease. *Ergo*... something important is hidden in the mucuna.

Obviously, no one can, at this point, "invent" *Mucuna pruriens* treatment as it has existed in India for thousands of years. Some, however, have patented certain techniques for extracting levodopa and other substances which are ingredients of these legumes. These physicians provide documentation in their patents which conclude that the use of these extracts of mucuna have advantages over the orthodox treatment with synthetic levodopa (Sinemet or Madopar).

And they aren't the only ones. Other prestigious neurologists (B.V. Manyam, S.C. Pruthi and others) have also recorded separate patents of mucuna extracts, with few variations. Mucuna must represent something important because everyone wants to endorse it.

One can assume that a there is a strong commercial competition in the running, and we can only hope that it will result in the benefit of patients.

DR. OLANOW AND DR. LEES

These two neurologists are almost legendary models for all those interested in Parkinson's disease.

C. Warren Olanow was educated at The University of Toronto and Columbia University and is now a professor at the Ichan School of Medince at Mount Sinai. He has served as president of the Movement Disorder Society and a member of the NASA Committee of Biomedical Research. He is the author of over 300 publications on Neurodegeneration and Parkinson's disease. In the last decade Olanow has been the most frequently cited researcher in the field.

Andrew Lees shows a hint of audacity and unorthodoxy in some of the topics he chooses: I remember with delight his lectures on "hedonistic homeostasis" (the internal balance of emotions and pleasure). So it did not surprise me to find that he is interested not only in new horizons for treatment of Parkinson's disease but also, in this case, Ayurveda herbs.

A more prudent and orthodox neurologist would probably have discarded such an idea, but Dr. Lees sensed its possibilities and advantages.

He is a Professor at National Hospital, Queen Square, London, he defined the criteria for the diagnosis of Parkinson's disease currently in use and he was the most cited researcher in this field around the world in 2011.

PATENTS OF EXTRACTS OF MUCUNA

The people who have proprietary over certain techniques of Mucuna extracts -WO 2004039385-A2 (86) and U.S. 7470441-B2- [37] are not amateurs.

Neurologists Lees and Olanow are world leaders in Parkinson's disease and I haveve seen them at many medical conventions. Of the remaining signers I recognize Hildebert Wagner, Editor for the *International Journal of Phytomedicine*. The fourth, R. van de Giessen, publishes articles related to the pharmaceutical industry.

These four researchers, a great team, have developed specific techniques to extract various substances from mucuna, not only levodopa. As they have detailed, many of the ingredients are indicated "*...for preventing, alleviating or treating neurological diseases*", for general use as "*a pharmaceutical combination for neuroprotection or neurostimulation*" and, more specifically, "*for the treatment of Parkinson's disease*". They have left little to chance.

ZANDOPA AND A COCKTAIL WITH MUCUNA

The previously mentioned Zandopa brand from Zandu Laboratories, which owns the patent for mucuna powder product known as HP-200, was used in important clinical trials [73] [87] and has been marketed for several years.

Som C. Pruthi has patented [88] a combination from the Ayurveda tradition that mainly contains mucuna (between 55 and 99%), together with *Piper longum* and *Zingiber officinalis*.

He described a woman diagnosed with Parkinson's at age 51 that did not tolerate conventional medicines. She took Pruthi's combination of mucuna for 12 years. In this long period it was found that progression of the disease was very slow, and side effects were not detected.

AN EXTRA-CONCENTRATED EXTRACT

The drawback of mucuna powder and primitive extracts is the large volume of legume one needs to consume in order to achieve sufficient blood levels of levodopa. This produces overeating and gastrointestinal upset, and causes many to abandon this therapy.

To avoid this trouble, Manyam has patented a method [89] involving the removal of grease from the cotyledons of the seeds. Using ethanol as a solvent, the concentrated extract is isolated, and finally freeze-dried.

With this technique, it is possible to process 2.5 kilograms (over 5 pounds) of mucuna powder, which is then reduced to just 46 grams (1.6 ounces). In this conversion the relative proportions of levodopa are maintained (or even increased). So the amount of vegetable to be ingested is reduced to less than 2%. In this way, it can be supplied as tablets, capsules or syrup; and even diluted for injection [89].

On the other hand, its efficacy has been demonstrated *in vitro* and in animals: when this concentrated extract is supplied to rats with "induced parkinsonism" their symptoms improve twice as much as compared to treatment with synthetic levodopa [76]. The advantages are significant.

MORE BENEFITS THAN CONVENTIONAL LEVODOPA

The foundations of the patent, based on the references provided, reveal that, in relation to standard levodopa-carbidopa medications (Sinemet) or levodopa-benserazide (Madopar), the extracts of mucuna have important advantages that confirm those listed in the previous chapter.

A WIDE THERAPEUTIC WINDOW

A therapeutic window is what we call the range of dosage in which a drug can be used without causing toxic effects, and this window is wider in mucuna. That means that there is a large margin between the minimally effective dose of mucuna and one that could cause damage in the body.

PATIENTS GET BETTER SOONER WITH MUCUNA

Researchers gave patients a tablet of Sinemet and they noticed the "on" effect after 54 minutes. But when they took mucuna they were already active after only 23-27 minutes. [26]

THE DURABLE EFFECT OF MUCUNA

In addition to being quick-acting, mucuna (at a dose of 30 grams) has been found to be effective for longer durations: patients were still "on" for 204 minutes after taking the seed extract, beating Sinemet tablet by half an hour [26].

LESS TOXIC THAN SYNTHETIC LEVODOPA

Neither acute nor chronic toxic effects have been described. Even with high doses of mucuna there were less adverse effects (nausea, abdominal discomfort) than in patients who received the equivalent of the conventional drugs [37].

Other long-term studies of mucuna (in monkeys and rats) have shown that the dreaded dyskinesia and other symptoms associated with continuous treatment with levodopa are lower, and in some cases even tend to improve. [33] [78]

COMBINATION THERAPY MAY BE DELAYED

This statement appears in the preamble of the documentation supporting the application for the patent. A professor of Phytotherapy and two neurologists believe that mucuna alone may suffice to relieve patients' symptoms for a period of time, and therefore combination therapy (levodopa plus agonists) can be delayed.

MUCUNA FOR ALMOST EVERYTHING

Mucuna seems to work for almost all diseases studied by neurologists. These renowned specialists believe that mucuna extracts may be useful in the treatment of multiple neurodegenerative processes.

Specifically, researchers have recorded the possibility of using extracts of mucuna for chorea, Parkinson's and Alzheimer's diseases, and vascular dementia [37]; further applications include many other metabolic disnutritive disorders and, systemic, endocrine and autoimmune disturbances (vitamin deficiency, lupus, demyelinating …), as well as neurotoxic, ischemic or traumatic injuries [86].

HIDDEN INGREDIENTS IN MUCUNA

Apart from levodopa, mucuna contains a variety of elements (as does the common bean). These are probably carbidopa-like substances (which inhibit decarboxylase), and others with a variety of characteristics.

A patient whose disease has evolved for several years knows that with the same dose of medication their symptoms may vary from time to time and that these changes are often not related to any specific factor. We also know that plasma levels of levodopa in Parkinson's patients vary depending on many factors (intestinal active transport, gastric emptying, competition in the blood-brain barrier, etc.).

With mucuna, fewer oscillations occur. It is assumed that it must contain certain substances that, in one or more respects, improve the effectiveness of levodopa, and even some components may act as dopamine agonists.

Further studies are needed to discover the hidden ingredients in mucuna which could be all or some of the following: carbidopa or other decarboxylase inhibitors; enzymes similar to entacapone or tolcapone; substances which promote intestinal motility and improve gastric emptying, thus accelerating the absorption of levodopa in the duodenum; or even amino acids that promote intestinal absorption or passage through the blood-brain barrier.

GRAY HAIR REVERSAL USING MUCUNA

Premature graying of hair is more frequent in Parkinson's patients, as there are complex relationships between melanin and dopamine.

Popular imagination considers gray hair to be a sign of suffering or a mark of premature aging [90] [91]. Classic and romantic novelists sensed this. Poe, for example, in his story *A Descent into the Maelström* in which the shipwrecked sailor relates how his hair turned gray and he became old in just one night from suffering.

It is surprising to see that in patients treated with mucuna, their gray hair regains its former darker color. This phenomenon has been described in a woman with whose white hair, after three months of treatment with mucuna, turned back to black [92], "like when I was young," she said. This is food for thought: the threads connecting youth, dopamine, suffering, old age, stress, and gray hair.

MUCUNA IS MORE THAN LEVODOPA

The available data has shown that *Mucuna pruriens* has special properties that distinguish it from synthetic levodopa. These data provide a basis for the patent registered by Olanow and Lees (quoted *verbatim*): "*the Mucuna pruriens formulation seems to possess potential advantages over existing commercially available synthetic L-Dopa formulations in that it combines a rapid onset of action with a comparable or longer duration of therapeutic response without increasing dyskinesias or acute LD toxicity in spite of much higher LD plasma levels...*" [37]

Natural ingredients (known or unknown) combined with levodopa may contribute to improvement of parkinsonian symptoms and reduction of dyskinesia [33][86]. This opens up the anticipation of important therapeutic progress and the hope of further studies to confirm that extracts of mucuna seeds are a safe and effective [33] alternative.

Currently, patients who are using mucuna under medical advice generally report a lowering of their doses of conventional drugs, and fewer side effects, in both the short and long term.

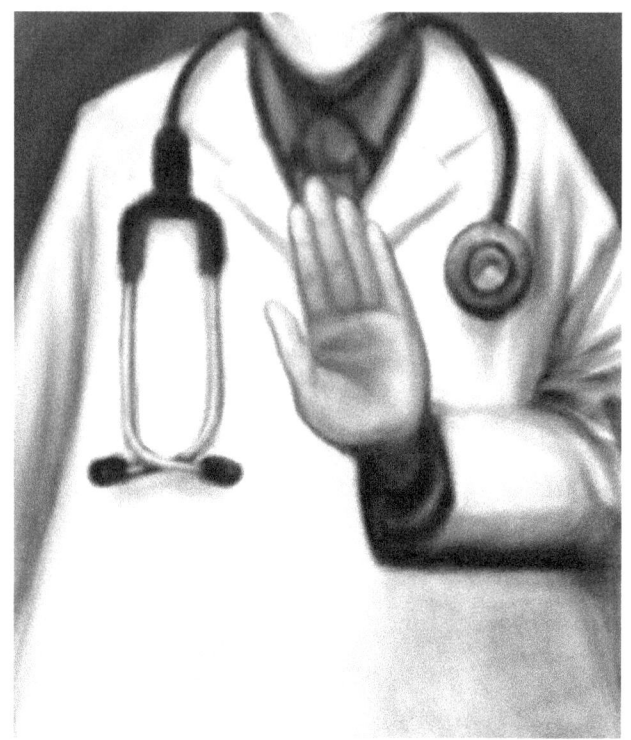

CONTRAINDICATIONS AND WARNINGS

Mucuna has general contraindications, similar to the synthetic levodopa. Other special situations in some patients need to be considered.

Always to be used under medical supervision.

7. Contraindications and warnings

Mucuna has some drawbacks. In principle, the levodopa in itself (albeit with other natural ingredients that improve tolerance) shares many of the contraindications and precautions applicable to synthetic levodopa. These warnings are well known and we will review some of them.

I want to begin by highlighting the main stumbling block to the beneficial use of mucuna: ignorance on the part of the patient and lack of medical information. A physician should monitor treatment at all times.

PATIENTS DO NOT KNOW WHAT THEY ARE TAKING

A major obstacle to treatment with mucuna is that patients don't have clear ideas about the drugs' intended purpose

They have heard of several cases where mucuna worked well, but usually these observations have come to them from people without any scientific knowledge, from non-professional websites or from commercial information intended for product sales.

Mucuna is sold freely on the Internet and many patients take it without medical supervision. Worse still, they engage in speculation based on bizarre opinions they encounter in the forums, and they absorb this erroneous information, and therefore lack sufficient knowledge to use it appropriately. However, occasionally patients are right or are very close to the truth, but there is still a danger of misuse. At times patients take mucuna simply because despair leads them to try anything.

THEY DESPISE WHAT THEY DO NOT KNOW

Many patients complain of the disdainful reaction they encounter when they ask their doctors about adding mucuna to their treatment regimen.

As it is an "unorthodox" therapy, it is perfectly understandable that the physician does not want to prescribe mucuna: it is not part of the generally accepted body of treatments they are trained to manage..

When a doctor decides to incorporate mucuna, he faces new difficulties, particularly with patients treated with other drugs. This requires the additional effort of studying the situation and designing a strategy for each individual case.

On the other hand, we cannot allow patients to treat themselves in hiding. Therefore, it is desirable that as doctors, we have to educate ourselves about mucuna so that we can choose to use it or not in a particular type of patient.

One should never despise the unfamiliar. After studying the properties of mucuna and weighing its advantages and disadvantages, we should decide on a rational basis, whether it is beneficial, neutral, or inadvisable for a specific case.

If the patient perceives that we master the subject, he will entrusted his care to us, rather than attempting to treat himself. That way, he will cooperate if we ban the mucuna or recommend a gradual dosage pattern. We earn their trust when we have enough information and credibility.

WHY ARE THERE NO FREQUENT MAJOR PROBLEMS?

Mucuna is not a placebo but, rather, has important effects. However anyone can buy it without a prescription, and most are taking it without medical supervision. These patients are not sufficiently familiar with the properties of mucuna, they do not know the side effects or complications that may arise; they do not take into account the interactions with other medications or the differences between individuals.

While this scenario suggests a public health issue, it fortunately does not usually cause serious problems. Why?

I think that one reason is the safety of the components of mucuna, which has been used for millennia in thousands or hundreds of thousands of patients in India without significant harmful effects.

Another issue is that the products are sold often in small doses as a dietary supplement. That is not, however, always the case: there are some preparations with excessive doses especially when combined with carbidopa (in Sinemet, Madopar or Stalevo), dopamine agonists or other antiparkinsonian drugs. It is necessary to use extreme caution.

CONTRAINDICATIONS OF LEVODOPA

Although better tolerated, mucuna contains a natural form of levodopa. In theory it should share the same contraindications, interactions and precautions of synthetic levodopa:

It is contraindicated in children, pregnancy and lactation (prolactin inhibition) and schizophrenia or psychosis.

It should be used with caution (and is best avoided) in cases of a medium to severe degree of heart disease or diabetes.

Do not take it with MAOIs, or with ergot.

Use caution (due to the additive effect) if the patient takes Levodopa (Sinemet, Madopar), COMT inhibitors (Entacapone Stalevo) or dopamine Agonists (rotigotine, pramipexole, ropinirole).

DRUGS THAT INTERACT WITH LEVODOPA

Neuroleptics antiemetics: metoclopramide (Reglan).

Neuroleptic antipsychotics.

Tetrabenazine. Baclofen.

Ayahuasca and other psychoanaleptics.

Nonselective MAOI (contraindicated).

Use caution with MAO-B; evaluate individual responses.

Anticholinergics. Dopamine uptake inhibitors.

Levodopa and beans (additive effect).

Ergot and other dopaminergics (additive effect).

Antihypertensives, antidepressants, sedatives, alpha blockers (prostate therapy): they may promote orthostatic hypotension.

Substances which inhibit the absorption of levodopa: spiramycin, salts of iron, antacids (dyspepsia).

SIDE EFFECTS WITH LEVODOPA

To avoid use in individuals with known allergy or hypersensitivity to *Mucuna pruriens* or components.

There have been some side effects of mucuna. In a study of patients with Parkinson's disease, a derivative of *Mucuna pruriens* caused minor adverse effects, which were mainly gastrointestinal in nature.

Isolated cases of acute toxic psychosis have been reported [93], probably due to levodopa content. Therefore, as with Sinemet and Madopar, its use should be avoided in patients with psychosis or schizophrenia

SPECIFIC WARNING ABOUT MUCUNA

We assume that all contraindications, interactions, precautions and side effects that we know about synthetic levodopa should be considered when taking levodopa from mucuna.

Specific contraindications include thinning of the blood (anticoagulants), and care should be taken with antiplatelet and anti-inflammatory drugs because mucuna increases clotting time.

Mucuna should not merge with anticoagulants (Sintrom, Dabigatran, heparin, warfarin) or with antiplatelet drugs such as clopidogrel. Caution should be exercised and the additive effect should be taken into account if it is associated with acetylsalicylic and NSAIDs (nonsteroidal anti-inflammatory).

We should also be careful with antidiabetic medicines: mucuna lows glycemic index, and thus is to be considered a potential additive effect. Other interactions are possible, so always consult your regular doctor.

On the one hand, it can be argued that mucuna has been used for many centuries in India and has been available for several years online without a prescription, and yet serious problems have not been revealed. But that is just an observation.

Regarding Sinemet and Madopar, we have thousands of controlled studies, while publications on mucuna are still scarce. One must therefore use greater caution when choosing mucuna. While the future appears to be positive, we need the confirmation of more scientific studies.

BE CAREFUL WHEN COMBINING MUCUNA AND GREEN TEA

Green tea enhances the effect of beans in general and of mucuna in particular. This effect can also be seen in patients taking Sinemet or Madopar: you should know this phenomenon due to the increase in potency it can cause.

There is something in green tea that acts like carbidopa. It contains polyphenols which inhibit dopa-decarboxylase [94], an action similar to that carried out by the carbidopa or benserazide contained in Sinemet or Madopar.

In addition, there is something that acts like entacapone in green tea. Ponifenol, EGCG (Epi-Gallo-Catecin-gallate) promotes the entry into the brain of levodopa and prolongs its bioavailability in the blood because it inhibits the COMT enzyme [95].

This action is similar to that of entacapone; namely beans mixed with green tea have Stalevo-like effects, but with different proportions. Obviously, if you take levodopa (mucuna or otherwise), its effectiveness will be reinforced and this should be taken into account as there is risk of overdose. Always consult your doctor.

These "carbidopa-like" and "entacapone-like" effects can be seen with green tea and they are independent of their other neuroprotective benefits [96] so the tea is recommended in many Parkinson's patients.

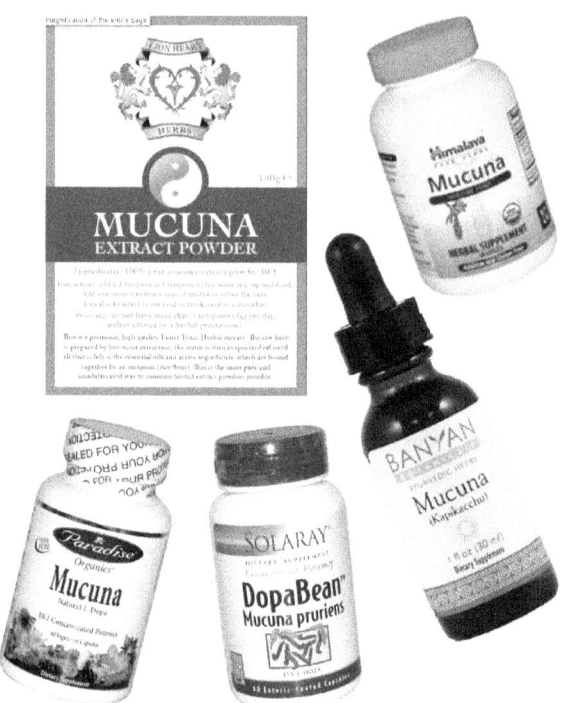

MANY PRODUCTS CONTAIN MUCUNA

In the market a variety of mucuna extracts are sold in powder, capsules or drops. Be careful with the different formulas and concentrations. You ought to know what you buy.

8. Dosage and presentations

To use mucuna correctly the premise is to be clear about what you want: it is simply a legume that contains levodopa naturally. Synthetic levodopa usually used in pharmaceutical preparations may be replaced in whole or in part by the levodopa contained in mucuna.

This sounds simple, but the point is that the dosages and concentrations can vary, so the guidelines must be individualized and, as we said, at present the patients (and even some doctors) lack sufficient information.

BEFORE USING MUCUNA

It is essential to find a neurologist who is interested in mucuna and who is adequately informed about this amazing plant and how it can influence the treatment of Parkinson's disease.

You should confirm everything with him and not conceal any information that may affect the treatment of your disease.

A STRATEGY TO START USING MUCUNA

First of all, ask your neurologist who knows your case. He can tell you if you can be treated with mucuna or not, based on your specific situation, the stage of your Parkinson's disease, and taking account other pathologies and conditions.

Secondly, your doctor will advise you on the purchase of the adequate formulation of mucuna depending on the dose administered.

It is prudent to start with low dose tablets and subsequently increase gradually; there is always time to increase the dosage.

Patience is key in the beginning: if you rush treatment for quick results, it is likely that you will experience some side effects which, although they are usually mild, can be bothersome. If the treatment proceeds too slowly on the other hand, you may think that the mucuna is not working and give up.

Third, adjustment the treatment: you almost always have to modify the dose and frequently have to remove some of the drugs previously prescribed (for Parkinson's disease or for your other pathologies).

CAREFUL WITH MISTAKES IN DOSAGE

There is no proven effective dose for mucuna. In clinical studies, some patients take 15 to 30 grams (half an ounce to one ounce) of mucuna preparation orally for a week, but I discourage such quantities, which I consider too high.

Any medication (which mucuna is) should be administered initially in small amounts, keeping in mind the particular case of the patient and the purpose of the treatment.

Doses of 15 and 30 grams of mucuna seed extract were used for a specific experiment, with strict medical check-ups, knowing well the formulation of the product and its origin, and taking into account many other factors.

The researchers work under controlled conditions: they select patients without contraindications and remove any incompatible drugs and other medications that may alter the absorption or metabolism of levodopa, etc.

That is not what happens when a patient buys mucuna just anywhere, and self-medicates with little information and without medical supervision.

BE CAREFUL WHEN BUYING MUCUNA

A consumer may purchase capsules of 200 mg of levodopa with a 15% concentration or 800 mg tablets with a 50% concentration, and these are two completely different products.

Sometimes patients have bought the product on eBay knowing nothing of their provider, and they receive a package whose content is not guaranteed and whose concentration is not safe. The patient then will then dilute the material in water without knowing how much to measure out.

Always use mucuna extracts that are dispensed by known, reliable suppliers. In the final chapter, we give a brief description of some of these.

PRICE SHOULD NOT MATTER AT THE BEGINNING

The price of mucuna, while not expensive, can be too much for some. That should be considered in the long-term as it could be in use for many months or years.

However, at first, the price does not matter much because the goal is to establish the dose for each patient. The main advice I give is to buy a product from a trusted brand and start with very low doses to be increased later.

In this first stage the daily cost will be minimal because the doses are low and the tablets or capsules have low concentrations of levodopa.

The important thing is to know if you feel better with mucuna. At this stage you should not buy any foreign preparation from distant countries through unknown sellers on eBay. Later, when we find the dose that fits a particular patient, then we can ultimately plan a more affordable product once we make sure that it is trustworthy.

PRESENTATIONS

There are so widely available that the Internet is flooded with numerous commercial offers.

I have selected some brands based on logical criteria: those with the longest history or best known, the most widely used, those that describe the content more clearly, and those coming from trusted providers.

In future editions of this book and its companion webpage (www.levodopa.net, www.parkinson-mucuna.com) I can offer an expanded and more precisely detailed catalogue of various formulations with different concentrations making for easier case-by-case adjustments.

Below is a summary of the presentations of mucuna grouped into seven sections.

a) **Mucuna powder**

b) **Mucuna in tinctures or concentrated extracts**

c) **Mucuna capsules or tablets, low dose** (15 to 30 mg of "real" natural levodopa), ideal to start taking mucuna.

d) **Mucuna in capsules or tablets, medium dose**

e) **Mucuna in capsules or tablets, high dose**

f) **Tincture or mucuna drops**

g) **Mucuna mixed with other substances**

There are many cheaper versions available, but I know their contents, and I have chosen prominent and accredited suppliers.

Among these, I prefer Anastore (with offices in Spain and France) and Amazon, which sells mucuna in France but not in Spain.

Other suppliers based in the United States (Amazon.com, iHerb) make the product more expensive due payment customs in countries in which it is available for purchase. At this point, these sources usually deny shipping to Spain. One option for the consumer in Spain would be to get it on eBay but you must be very sure about the provider.

a) Mucuna powder

The classic presentation is powder from mucuna seeds. It is very bothersome to prepare as the powder must be diluted in water or other liquid (not milk because it hinders absorption). It has a very unpleasant taste that laboratories try to hide by sweetening it.

The great advantage is the ability to adjust the exact for smaller doses that are always recommended at the beginning. In countries (such as Spain) where it is more difficult to find capsules or tablets with small doses, one may start with mucuna powder. There are many brands offered, but here I describe only the original, which is sent directly from India.

ZANDOPA HP-200.

This drug was marketed in India after the publication of an innovative study in Parkinson's patients in which an average of 6 sachets (+ -3) of mucuna seed powder (7.5

grams with levodopa 250 mg, i.e. 3.3%) were administered to each patient.

I would like to emphasize that this mucuna levodopa dose is relatively high (1,500 milligrams), especially for those who had never taken levodopa, and if combined with one or two tablets of Sinemet there is an obvious risk of overdose.

Other than those patients, there were no problems probably because this natural levodopa is not combined with carbidopa (as in Sinemet).

In theory the levodopa from mucuna, as it lacks carbidopa, should be removed rapidly from the blood... unless the plant contains other ingredients to avoid it.

After taking the mucuna powder (dissolved in water), blood levels of levodopa behave similarly to those observed with the synthetic version of levodopa. The difference is that the maximum dose does not show as marked an effect [87], and clinical efficacy is similar or greater.

COMMON MISTAKES IN PRESCRIBING ZANDOPA

Equivalences of Zandopa powder are administered to people who take only levodopa (without carbidopa), something which hardly occurs in the West, so that errors are very common.

According to the manufacturer every measure of mucuna powder (7.5 grams) is equivalent to 250 mg of synthetic levodopa. But this is only when the patient does not take carbidopa at all. However, almost all patients mix mucuna powder with some Sinemet or Stalevo in which case it is necessary to assume that the carbidopa is working.

The equivalence for Zandopat is not clear to the uninitiated. If you follow the laboratoy indications you must give 30 grams of powder to replace the Sinemet 25/250 tablet (4 small cups).

This is the ratio that was used in the original study, but in practice it is too high and can cause side effects (nausea, vomiting, and malaise) so I do not recommend it.

The dosage is individualized and you have to start with small, adequately spaced doses.

The laboratory has verified this and thus expressed it in the brochure, although not sufficiently emphasized.

b) Mucuna in very low doses (15-30 mg)

We said that it is highly recommended to start with low doses of mucuna in order to discern a suitable treatment for each case and situation. Therefore, I suggest starting with presentations of very low amounts of mucuna, for example, rather than those listed principally to treat the Parkinson's disease, those that are sold with general indications as "tonics", aphrodisiacs or "revitalizers".

HIMALAYA

This brand is promoted as a "nerve tonic." It comes in a capsule of 250 mg of mucuna extract 6% which is equivalent to 15 mg of pure levodopa.

Currently, this product only appears on the web pages of the United Sates and is not sent to Spain.

ADVANCE PHYSICIAN

Mucuna extract comes in 200 mg capsules with no concentration indicated on the label, which usually means it is low (15% or less).

This is not shipped to Spain either.

c) Mucuna in low doses (50-60 mg)

These are available in Spain through Andorra and France. I highlight three brands here.

SOLARAY DOPA-BEAN

Sold as a dietary supplement, without specifying that it is used to treat Parkinson's disease.

Each capsule contains 333 mg of extract of the *Mucuna pruriens* (velvet beans) seed in a concentration of 15%, which is 50 mg of natural levodopa (equivalent to the synthetic levodopa in half a tablet of Sinemet Plus or one fifth of Sinemet 250). It is a good choice to start with. Some pharmacies sell this online in Andorra.

AYURVANA MUCUNA

Very similar to the previous one, it contains 370 mg of extract of mucuna 15% which translates to 55 mg of natural levodopa. You can order it on Amazon France.

BONUSAN

These are vegetable capsules with mucuna 400mg 15%, i.e. 60 mg of levodopa. It is another French product available through Andorra but is also provided by a pharmacy in Barcelona, and recently, a leading e-commerce company delivered some in less than 4 days (see Chapter 12).

d) Mucuna in medium doses (75-100 mg)

I will mention two brands, both of which can be obtained through the French web page of Amazon. They contain significant doses and thus it is highly recommended that it be prescribed and controlled by a doctor.

VITAWORLD

Capsules of 500 mg mucuna 15%, about 75 milligrams of levodopa.

ANASTORE

This mucuna preparation is possibly the easiest to obtain in our country, because the supplier has a Spanish delegation able to import the product from France.

It contains 100 mg of natural levodopa (the same as a tablet of Sinemet Plus) in a capsule of 200 milligrams of extract of mucuna which is quite concentrated (50%).

BIOVEA MUCUNA DOPA

Recently available, you can now buy it from Spain and almost anywhere in the world. Each capsule has 250 mg mucuna seed extract 40% equivalent to 100 mg of levodopa.

e) Mucuna in high doses (more than 100 mg)

These are advisable only when the doctor has already adjusted the daily dose for the patient.

NOW DOPA MUCUNA

These capsules are large because it contains 120 mg of levodopa and, as it is a low concentration (15%), 800 mg of powdered seeds are needed.

It is sold in France and can be ordered online.

f) Tincture or Mucuna drops

These are difficult to buy, their concentrations are often too high, and it is more troublesome to establish the dosage unless you are an expert. I don't recommend it.

g) Mucuna mixed with other substances

Some theories assert that there are people with a relative nutritional deficiency or imbalance of certain precursor amino acids of dopamine and serotonin [97], and that this causes or worsens Parkinson's disease, depression and other related disorders involving centrally acting monoamines.

In this vein, some have proposed mucuna combined with tyrosine, tryptophan and others to relieve this imbalance of amino acids. This theory, enthusiastically promoted by Dr. M. Hinz [98], recommends products that combine levodopa with tryptophan, tyrosine, cysteine and cofactors in order to recuperate the balance.

These treatments can be useful, and future studies are needed to expand on the effect of amino acids and other nutritional aspects of Parkinson's disease and their influence on the behavior of levodopa.

There is some progress in treatment from that angle, but it is not yet confirmed and results can be highly variable.

So far I do not recommend the combined preparations as some do, mixing tyrosine, green tea (carbidopa action exerted a slight), lipoic acid, ginseng, ginkgo, etc. It will suffice to adjust the dosage of mucuna.

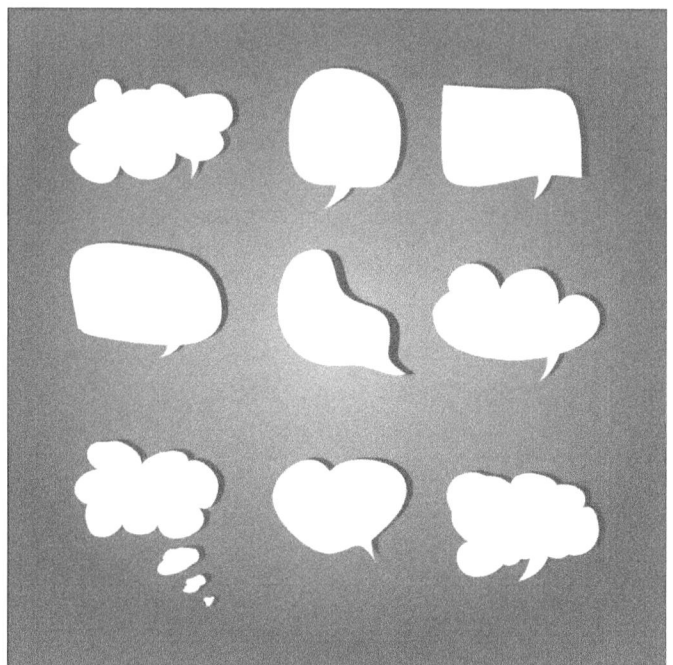

MUCUNA IN INTERNET FORUMS

They know that mucuna works, but lack general information and doctors do not usually help much.

In Forum the patients are looking for the answers that doctors do not give in clinical consultations.

9. Testimonials from those who take mucuna

During the initial consultation with the patient, to encourage him to talk, I say: *I know more about Parkinson's disease than you, but when it comes to "your Parkinson's", your discomfort throughout the day and how the medicines make you feel, you know much more than I.*

I have learned a lot from patients, they are our best book, and I have taken in what they tell me: "*Conjectures of a neurologist who listened to a thousand Parkinson's patients*" (R. González Maldonado, 2014).

In Spain mucuna is still little used, and my practical experience is limited, so I have read, I have studied and I have compared patients who are discussed in various forums in Europe and North America. I summarize here some of my conclusions.

FORUMS ON MUCUNA

Reviews on mucuna are common in Parkinson's disease forums. These are interesting because they illustrate specific situations in different people using extracts combined with conventional drugs.

I give you a few examples with the caveat that these are subjective opinions of people without medical knowledge, and should not be imitated; they are only expressing their experiences:

http://www.iocob.nl/english-articles/mucuna-pruriens-for-parkinsons-disease.html

http://www.blog.parkinsonsrecovery.com/category/mucuna

http://neurotalk.psychcentral.com/archive/index.php/t-48015.html

I invite the reader to attend those interesting forums and also to participate, as a curiosity. Keep in mind that there individual cases of people (who usually have no medical knowledge) are related. These views are not filtered and can cause errors. You are always obliged to consult a doctor.

CONCLUSIONS DERIVED FROM THESE FORUMS

To write this book I found useful and inspiring numerous data extracted from forums where Parkinson's patients relate their experiences with mucuna.

These comments, and other, more incisive testimonials not reproduced here, generally reflect a mixture of hope and despair.

Sometimes they attack doctors and the pharmaceutical industry. They even suggest that some form of passivity is allied with economic interests.

They claim that it is essential that well-controlled clinical trials be conducted to discover in depth the true properties of mucuna in order to improve the treatment of Parkinson's disease.

I hope this book can help achieve that goal.

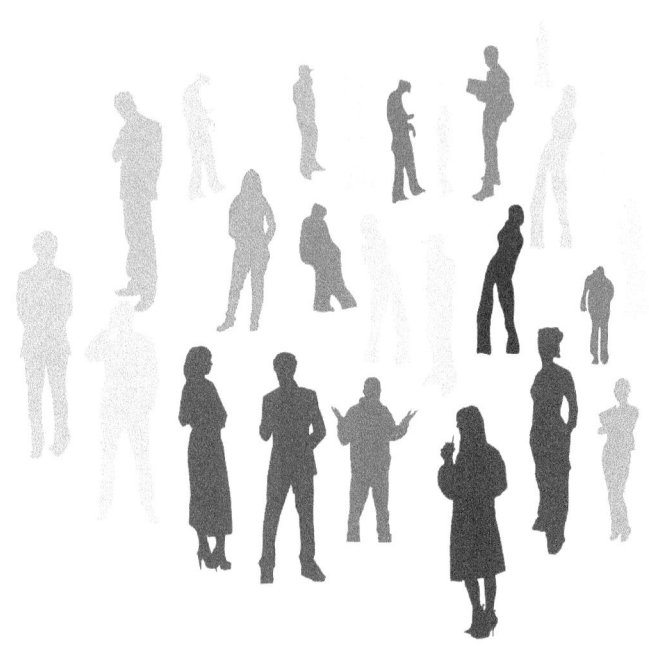

PRACTICE IN EACH CASE IS DIFFERENT

To start with mucuna, the strategy is different in each case, those who have never taken levodopa, those with levodopa-carbidopa-entacapone, or selegiline or using agonists, different developmental stage, medical contraindications...

10. How to start taking mucuna: case studies

I reiterate: although I try to substantiate my convictions, I expose in these pages my personal opinions about mucuna, which therefore are open to debate. Furthermore, I do not take responsibility for direct application of any treatment. Rather, patients must always consult their regular doctors before acting on any medical advice.

The guidelines I give here on the use of mucuna are always of a general nature, are indicative and should then be applied to the specific clinical situation of the individual patient. Under this premise, I will present some case studies.

MUCUNA IS NOT FOR EVERYONE

Mucuna is a good supplementary treatment in some patients with Parkinson's disease, but is not indicated in all cases.

This discrepancy might be due not only to possible side effects, which fortunately are usually few, but because it is not useful in certain stages of the disease.

AN INCREASE IN MUCUNA MEANS A DECREASE IN PHARMACEUTICAL DRUGS

In the majority of patients, mucuna must be combined (according to medical criteria) with other antiparkinsonian drugs. In some cases, especially at the beginning, this may be the only treatment.

It is advisable (under supervision) to add mucuna slowly while gradually decreasing the doses of Sinemet or other conventional antiparkinsonian drugs [99].

The ultimate goal is for the patient to feel better as he takes fewer prescription drugs and suffers fewer side effects to boot. These are the findings of a review of extensive and detailed literature [99].

NOT FOR PEOPLE WITHOUT PARKINSON'S DISEASE

Mucuna should not be used as a preventive treatment for Parkinson's disease. Although it has fewer side effects than synthetic levodopa, mucuna is a "drug" and should not be used previous to the onset of the disease.

PARKINSON'S DIAGNOSIS UP TO 55 YEARS

In a young person, diagnosed prior to the age of 60, orthodox treatment aims to delay as long as possible the use of levodopa (Sinemet, Madopar, Stalevo). Instead, it is currently used rasagiline (Azilect) or dopamine agonists such as pramipexole (Mirapex), rotigotine (Neupro patches) or ropinirole.

Later, when levodopa becomes necessary, the patient and his doctor can take into consideration the option of starting with mucuna because it causes less long term dyskinesia. It is a decision that must be shared by doctor and patient.

Although rasagiline and selegiline are MAO-B (incomplete), as a precaution it is preferable to stop taking them two weeks before starting the mucuna.

If the patient also received treatment with dopamine agonists the doctor may want to reduce those as well.

In any case, mucuna would be taken in very low doses (200 mg of formulas 15 %) at first, and then would gradually be increased.

PARKINSON'S DIAGNOSIS AT 75 YEARS-OLD

When the symptoms first appear after age 70, the treatment strategy changes. Usually when Parkinson's disease starts late it is more benign and treatment is simplified.

Moreover, in these older patients, the premise is to rule out the possibility of cardiac or other general problems, and to prevent any possible interactions with medications currently in use. At that age I would rather avoid dopamine agonists and by prescribing low doses of levodopa to gradually be increased.

If you opt for the mucuna, you must start with very low doses (200 mg formulas 15%) and then move up progressively. You can later try to improve the bioavailability of levodopa by adding some carbidopa.

Tablets containing only carbidopa (Lodosyn) are sold in some countries. In Spain carbidopa is not available independently. In these cases you can resort to adding Sinemet Plus (which has a higher proportion of carbidopa). We are providing 12.5 mg of carbidopa with half of a tablet. However, this tablet also contains 50 mg of synthetic levodopa thus it would be necessary to deduct a portion of the dose of mucuna (the equivalent of natural levodopa).

For example, you can start by adding half of a tablet of Sinemet Plus per 100-150 mg while removing one tablet of 800 mg Mucuna 15%, continuing the remaining medications.

TRIALS WITH SINEMET-FREE PATIENTS

In practice, almost all patients with Parkinson's disease will be treated at some point in their lives with the synthetic levodopa in Sinemet, Madopar or Stalevo.

We found that some of our patients had not yet used these drugs. This is usually due to one of two factors: they are either in the early stages of the disease or, even if they have been diagnosed for months or years, they are young (under 60 years) and the doctor opted to delay the use of synthetic levodopa for fear of later complications (dyskinesia and others).

On the other hand patients may have been fortunate enough to have maintained a good functional capacity, and have not yet needed agonists or other antiparkinsonian drugs.

These patients who never used synthetic levodopa (Sinemet, Madopar or Stalevo) are potential candidates for testing the response to levodopa with natural extracts of mucuna seed.

In the course of the disease there is a specific time in which the doctor decides to start treating with levodopa (which is the most effective treatment). At that point, common sense suggests that the natural form of levodopa is a legitimate choice instead of the synthetic form.

Treatment should be started with seed extracts of mucuna in low-concentration formulas (15%) in small amounts. With these low doses the symptoms still may not have improved but we have established that mucuna is well tolerated. From there, we must increase dosage gradually according to patient response.

PATIENTS TAKING LOW DOSES OF SINEMET

If a patient has been on a very low dose of Sinemet (or Madopar), 100 to 300 milligrams a day, for a short period of time, the doctor may consider gradually changing to mucuna extracts, other circumstances permitting.

The strategy is to gradually remove the synthetic levodopa while mucuna is added. But the problem is more complex for carbidopa (or benserazide) which is also contained in these tablets.

If the functional status of the patient is satisfactory and he is on a very low dose of Sinemet (or Madopar), it is even possible to dispense these drugs. It is worth enduring a short period of minor clinical deterioration, so that the patient is left without any drugs before starting mucuna.

PATIENTS TAKING A MEDIUM DOSE OF SINEMET

Commonly, people who are taking synthetic levodopa (especially if the dose is medium or high) cannot do without it if it is reduced rapidly, not least because is associated with carbidopa (or benserazide).

In these cases one can use half a tablet of Sinemet 25/100 Plus (better than 25/250 Sinemet), to provide a bit of carbidopa (12.5 mg), since it includes some synthetic levodopa (50 mg) which logically should be considered in addition to the natural levodopa provided by mucuna.

At this point, a problem arises for the neurologist: mucuna levodopa is approximately three times more potent than the synthetic version, but that relationship changes when carbidopa is added to one or the other.

When you read the prospectuses of mucuna preparations you can see recommendations of dosage that apply only to patients who take simply mucuna. The laboratory assumes that you are not taking carbidopa. But if you take carbidopa (due to a combined treatment of mucuna with Sinemet), then the amount of product recommended will contain too much levodopa.

Another point of confusion comes from clinical trials comparing Sinemet and mucuna extracts containing just natural levodopa without carbidopa (although the plant can provide similar but unknown substances with a milder effect). They employ an amount of mucuna with relatively high doses of levodopa (without carbidopa) to compare the clinical efficacy of the latter with respect to Sinemet.

Last but not least, we must take into account the idiosyncrasies of the patient: some react to mucuna sooner or more effectively, others experience weak or delayed responses.

This issue is complex and cooperation between the patient the neurologist in a supportive atmosphere is essential, choosing the best strategy at this juncture is a true example of the art of medicine.

Fortunately, the experience does not show major problems despite the chaos usually surrounding mucuna: freely permitted online without a prescription, patients' lack of knowledge, and the detachment most doctors feel regarding this topic. Under these conditions one would expect hundreds of medical complications to have been registered, and so far, I have heard of none.

PATIENTS TAKING STALEVO

In theory one could also replace some of the synthetic levodopa in Stalevo for the equivalent of mucuna levodopa (assuming that one would have to modify the proportions).

However, we would have to address all the issues raised in the previous section regarding Sinemet (because of its carbidopa content) along with the added problem of entacapone: since it inhibits COMT, the efficiency of mucuna levodopa is increased further, and the result is less predictable.

On the internet forums some of the most common complaints are discussed among those taking Stalevo along with the legume.

I have not heard of clinical studies comparing mucuna and Stalevo (levodopa + carbidopa + entacapone). So, while it is not as good, I suggest that if the patient and doctor agree, as a first step, Stalevo (at least some) would be replaced by the equivalent Sinemet and, as a second step, the issue could be addressed as detailed in the previous section.

TAKING RASAGILINE PLUS SINEMET

With the exception of some particular cases, selegiline has been displaced by rasagiline, which has a similar but more specific action.

Both are inhibitors of MAO (monoamine oxidase) type B enzyme which, inter alia, results in more effective brain dopamine.

It seems also that rasagiline and selegiline are neuroprotective, and therefore recommended from the beginning of the illness, especially in young people. These drugs can bring about a slight amelioration of motor symptoms.

In later stages of the disease and in older patients the rasagiline (or selegiline) complicates treatment. Remarkably, it increases adverse effects (hypotension and dyskinesia) when combined with Stalevo (carbidopa + levodopa + entacapone) without providing clear advantages over a Stalevo-only treatment, and achieving little benefit in relation to a Sinemet-only therapy [100].

Too many enzymes result inhibited: carbidopa restrains dopa-decarboxylase, entacapone slows down catechol-ortho-methyl-transferase, and rasagiline (or selegine) inactivates monoamine oxidase.

To make matters worse, sometimes this treatment is further associated with an antidepressant that prevents the reuptake of serotonin. In such cases complications are disseminated throughout the cerebral dopamine metabolism.

Common sense, or simple intuition, if you will, dictate my desire to flee from an artifice such as this.

Both selegiline and rasagiline are not absolute contraindications, and there is no firm theoretical basis to suspect this, but I suggest they be removed if one is planning to use mucuna.

In my opinion, the supposed benefits of combining mucuna with rasagiline and levodopa is mild and should be avoided, at least until further case studies are available.

PATIENTS WHO ONLY TAKE RASAGILINE

In young patients it is customary to delay the initiation of levodopa (Sinemet or Madopar), using instead rasagiline (or selegiline). For the one to two years that patients are on this drug, they remain levodopa "virgins".

As I mentioned before, it would be prudent to remove the Azilect (rasagiline) or Eldepryl (selegiline) before starting mucuna.

However, if patients are suddenly deprived for several days of a drug that had previously been useful, then they may complain of clinical deterioration during that period.

My proposal is to start testing the response to very low doses of "synthetic" levodopa combined with carbidopa (or benserazide): half of a tablet of Sinemet Plus (or a quarter of Madopar), equivalent to 50 mg of levodopa with its proportion of carbidopa (or benserazide).

Meanwhile, we must reduce the rasagiline (or selegiline) for several days before eliminating it.

Thus, on those days when patients are on half of a tablet of Sinemet Plus, their motor symptoms should not worsen, and, more importantly, we know how they tolerate "normal" levodopa.

An added advantage is that adverse effects are minimal or non-existent because carbidopa (or benserazide) eliminates peripheral cardiovascular and intestinal action.

As a second step, Sinemet (or Madopar) is replaced by low doses of mucuna as described in the corresponding section.

PATIENTS TAKING ONLY DOPAMINE AGONISTS

This group is large. Usually levodopa therapy is delayed in patients diagnosed before age 60, for fear of later complications. It is instead replaced with dopamine agonists that usually provide a good functional state for one to five years.

In general, if the daily amount of agonist is small, there would be minimal adverse effects to starting with mucuna. If the patient is already taking a medium or high amount of agonist, the neurologist should adjust the dose accordingly.

Patients treated with dopamine agonists have a tendency towards orthostatic hypotension which must be taken into account when adding levodopa, whether natural or synthetic.

The specific type of agonist is very important. Rotigotine (Neupro patches) is one of my favorite agonists. In theory, if there are no contraindications, and if under medical supervision, the patches can be combined with mucuna.

However, I have not yet found any publication that describes this association, perhaps this will be forthcoming in the near future.

Studies have been published describing patients treated with pramipexole (Mirapex) or Ropirinole who have received high doses of mucuna, and no significant adverse effects were observed.

Therefore it seems that in these patients previously treated with Mirapex or Ropirinole if mucuna were recommended, it could begin with low doses and slowly progress, always under the supervision of a neurologist.

In order to initiate the mucuna, the doctor may decide to slightly reduce the dose of agonist.

PATIENTS WHO TAKE AMANTADINE

Amantadine was originally a medicine used to treat influenza. It also acts as a partial dopamine agonist with special features and which became fashionable as a treatment in some Parkinson's patients who were unresponsive to other drugs. It is also assumed to be useful against dyskinesia.

In clinical trials patients treated with amantadine have received large doses of mucuna without encountering any significant adverse effects. However, if one is going to use mucuna, I recommend minimizing any substances that could interact with it.

Amantadine usually loses its effectiveness over time and it may be that the patient no longer needs the drug. If amantadine is not essential, it is preferable to remove it (gradually) before initiating mucuna.

PATIENTS TAKING STALEVO AND RASAGILINE

I do not advise mucuna in combination with Stalevo and rasagiline, at least initially.

It is common sense to note that this combination blends many enzyme inhibitors: monoamine oxidase (rasagiline or selegiline), COMT catechol-ortho-methyl-transferase (entacapone) and decarboxylase (carbidopa).

All neurologists see patients that combine levodopa, carbidopa, entacapone and rasagiline, but this quartet usually produces more problems [100] than it solves. That is also my own experience and I avoid that situation when I can.

To test mucuna in these cases, I recommend first removing the rasagiline. As a second step you can follow the protocol that I have mentioned in the section on Stalevo.

PATIENTS WHO TRIED APOMORPHINE

There is no publication describing experiences with the use of mucuna in patients treated with apomorphine.

On the other hand, when a patient requires this drug (by injector pen or infusion pump) the disease is very advanced and the expectations of improvement with mucuna are minimal. I do not advise it.

POLYPHARMACY AND MANY YEARS OF PARKINSON'S

Often, after many years of suffering from Parkinson's disease, patients turn to velvet beans (or other supposedly miraculous techniques) searching for any remedy as a last resort. Those are precisely the cases where it is less desirable to use mucuna.

Once the disease is already very advanced, there are many other important drugs that cannot be removed from the treatment plan, and if the general condition of the patient is poor, this is not the time to do "experiments".

In some specific cases, this can be tried using isolated doses of mucuna during the "off" periods, in an attempted "rescue" when there is little to lose. However, the physician must weigh the relationship between expected benefit and possible interactions.

WHEN PATIENTS TAKE OTHER DRUGS

Patients with multiple diagnoses or who are taking many medications should avoid mucuna.

There are some contrasting interactions as well as the possibility of other yet unknown effects.

I discourage the use of mucuna in these cases until more clinical trials are available.

MUCUNA ONLY AS THE "RESCUE" DOSE

This possibility makes sense. In patients who have had Parkinson's disease for many years and have been taking various medications, the option of taking mucuna may be considered as an extra and occasional aid, when they begin to suffer the "off" period.

There was a patient comment to this effect on the forum, that I picked up in chapter 9, subsection *About mucuna occasionally*.

ADDING CARBIDOPA TO MUCUNA

Synthetic levodopa in Sinemet is improved by carbidopa. This increases its clinical efficacy and prevents peripheral side effects (nausea, tachycardia).

Carbidopa further improves mucuna: it reduces the already mild side effects and makes it two or three times stronger.

This effect should be taken into account when a patient combines mucuna and Sinemet (or Madopar or Stalevo). These drugs contain carbidopa, which will also act with mucuna levodopa making it more effective (so it will be necessary to reduce the theoretical dose).

What happens if one is not taking Sinemet or other drugs? Then mucuna levodopa may be insufficient.

This group of patients is complaining that the mucuna "does nothing" and the reason is that levodopa is removed rapidly from the blood by the decarboxylase before it can reach the brain.

The solution: mucuna may be combined with carbidopa which in some countries is sold separately (this is called Lodosyn).

And what if you cannot buy Lodosyn? There is the option of taking half of a tablet of Sinemet Plus: 12.5 mg carbidopa including 50 mg of synthetic levodopa. This amount will be subtracted from the previous dose of levodopa from mucuna, bearing in mind that it will now be more potent.

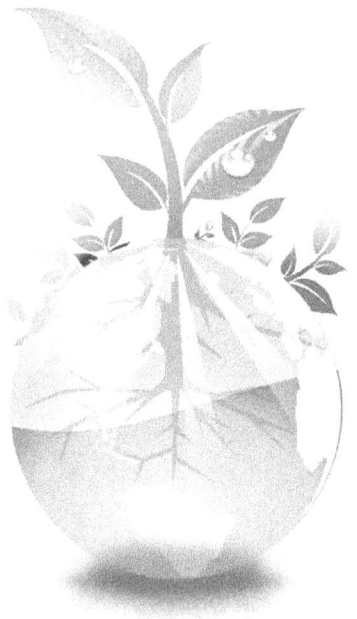

THE FUTURE OF MUCUNA

We expect that new clinical trials will confirm the efficacy of Mucuna to treat many patients with Parkinson's disease. It seems that natural levodopa is more effective and has less side effects in the short and long term.

11. The future of mucuna

To discuss the future of the mucuna we must first know what the holders of patents for extracts have in mind, and how the pharmaceutical industry plans to support them.

In Internet forums some patients speculate suspicions and express opinions that I do not share. I do not think that there is an attempt to "park" the development of natural levodopa since it can provide so many benefits to patients.

Natural levodopa from mucuna, as well as being very affordable (this plant is difficult to eradicate once established), is more effective and less toxic than the synthetic levodopa currently sold. So it would be inhuman not to foster research about it.

Why, then, in the ten years since the first patent was registered have researchers not kept up with the necessary studies? The situation is reminiscent of the story of the Spanish comedy *El perro del hortelano* (The orchard owner's dog), who neither eats nor lets others eat.

I have not found any explanation by neurologists nor any laboratory involved in this topic.

Qui prodest? This classical Latin quotation is heard in the films of detectives that are looking for a culprit: Who benefits if there is no new research?

Meanwhile adequate clinical trials using mucuna remain almost clandestine, and are based on limited experiences without adequate controls. To establish general rules for the use of natural levodopa, we need rigorous testing protocols that provide a reasonable foundation of data, but so far we are limited to mere conjectures and personal experiences.

Levodopa was discovered as a result of Gugenheim's bean eating binge. It is known that beans contain natural levodopa (better than the synthetic version), and that it is highly concentrated in beans growing in the tropics as mucuna. I hope, for the sake of the many patients who need it, that there will soon to be progress in this area.

CARBIDOPA AND AMINO ACIDS

The profile of enzymes looks different in each patient: some feel better with carbidopa and others prefer benserazide. In addition, there may be other inhibitors of the decarboxylase (in mucuna or other sources) that may be suitable for some.

In the same way, different amino acids and nutrients interact differently with each type of levodopa (synthetic or natural) in an unknown manner, but we know that they influence its bioavailability and clinical efficacy. It is a field of research in which progress is being made.

MUCUNA: THE LEVODOPA FOR THE POOR

In Africa and the Caribbean I have seen Parkinson's patients in a very deteriorated state, who are not treated with levodopa because they are unable to afford Sinemet, Madopar or Stalevo. Neither they nor their governments can bear this expense.

Ironically in their countries levodopa is everywhere, mucuna grows spontaneously and spreads so fast that they even have to pull up it so it does not invade other crops.

The plant contains a large amount of levodopa, a treasure trove for those patients in the third world. Ailing inhabitants need this levodopa to live better and longer. It is outrageously unfair.

A recent study (MDS World Congress in Stockholm. June 2014) [101] offered an option: use of mucuna levodopa is very accessible in countries that cannot afford Sinemet, Madopar or Stalevo.

NEUROLOGISTS IN GHANA AND ZAMBIA

I applaud the laudable deeds of neurologists who have opened clinics for patients in Ghana and Zambia where they have already served over 100 patients.

There they cannot prescribe Sinemet because it costs a prohibitive dollar and a half each day per patient, meanwhile *Mucuna pruriens* grows spontaneously all around them.

With the collaboration of the local authorities, they began to systematically prepare seeds of mucuna (harvesting 12 different types) cooking them first to eliminate anti nutritive substances.

They administered mucuna without special extraction methods, although they could not integrate carbidopa, and have obtained the first results: the levels of levodopa in the blood increase, demonstrating that it is being absorbed [101] [102].

Patients improved although the system is so primitive that they suffered some side effects such as nausea, dry mouth, and orthostatic hypotension. [102]

IT IS RIGHT TO STUDY THIS OPTION

The initiative of these pioneers of mucuna treatment in Africa is promising. However, this situation must be regulated. Who could ever infringe on such an important humanitarian effort?

Studies of mucuna in Parkinson's disease should be expanded. Inexpensive levodopa should be provided to patients with few resources in poor countries. It could be that doctors and patients of the West ... finally imitate the less fortunate.

WHY IS IT SO EXPENSIVE IN THE WEST?

Mucuna is very cheap but extracts in the West cost more than the Sinemet or Madopar, not least because in many countries the only possibility is to buy it online. Being a plant that grows vigorously and even invasively it is hard to understand why in the West it is so expensive when used in effective doses.

Cost also depends on the specific preparation and where it is purchased. I have done calculations by number of capsules, content and price. The variations are monumental. The cost of one gram of levodopa (10 tablets of Sinemet Plus) contained in extracts of mucuna ranges between 1 and 15 euros (one brand is fifteen times more expensive than the other!).

WHY IS MUCUNA NOT PRESCRIBED BY NEUROLOGISTS?

First, neurologists do not consider it a fully approved drug marketed as a medicine (although Zandopa is itself registered as such). And that is one explanation for not prescribing it. Further, it is not subsidized by the public health system. What is harder to understand is why doctors often refuse to discuss mucuna with their patients.

Another explanation is the lack of time available for each patient visit and the fact that doctors are exasperated by the typical patient who comes in asking about a long list of "things he has read on the internet."

In addition, and I do not know why, the necessary clinical studies on such a promising treatment have not advanced further.

There is one more justification: according to available data, it is currently difficult to decipher the true value of mucuna as an add-on option in Parkinson's disease.

Doses, concentrations and conversions are somewhat complicated in practice. So the norm is to follow the patterns established by official protocols. My personal opinion is that we are delaying the foreseeable benefits of mucuna.

MUCUNA AND OTHER PLANTS

Strategies for the future treatment of Parkinson's disease are vast and varied.

As an aspect of the subject of this book I want to emphasize that future treatments will include the search for nutritional factors influencing the development of Parkinson's disease as well as research leading to the discovery of new bioactive compounds in plants and phyto-derivatives.

Mucuna seems to be a fundamental part of this horizon. As an example, it seems paradigmatic, read in the following paragraph a personal account of a Parkinson's patient who has a degree in chemistry.

CHEMISTRY PROFESSOR PREPARES HIS MUCUNA

The president of the Parkinson's Society of India, D. Deo is a chemist and suffers from the disease. With the help of a colleague, he prepares his own mucuna extracts that he has been taking for several years.

A conference presented his experience which I reproduce *verbatim*:

"As an experimental project, I started using naikurna (Mucuna pruriens) and within days it stabilized my movements. Gradually, I could reduce 70% of my daily dose of levodopa–carbidopa and began to feel better".

"Consumption of natural levodopa as naikurna powder has, in my case, never caused any side-effects".

"The only disadvantage is the need to take large quantities of the powder. A leading chemist helped me isolate levodopa by the solvent extraction method and over the past 2 years this liquid has had encouraging results".

"I think it has helped me stop progression of my disease. I presented my experience at a meeting of the Parkinson's Disease Association after which many patients came forward to try this natural medicine and have now acknowledged its benefits".

"I provide free naikurna (mucuna pruriens) extract to the needy. The Parkinson's Disease Association helped me get in touch with the leading neurologists in India. They have taken a keen interest in my efforts to spread the use of this complementary medicine".

"My intention in its propagation is based on two beneficial aspects. It substantially reduces the cost of medicines—is a great boon to the large number of poor patients in India— and more importantly, it provides relief with no side effects".[77]

PATIENTS CAN HELP A LOT

People with Parkinson's are usually intelligent observers, are well informed about the disease and, especially, are very aware how they fare with the different treatments.

The experience of patients, including their views (which can then be relativized for general benefit) and their subjective impressions of the effects of a treatment in particular, are very important assets to keep us learning about Parkinson's disease.

I have learned a lot by listening to these patients, and I pride myself on it. I suggest you ask your doctor his impression about what you can expect from mucuna.

I also encourage you to comment on the forums by, rather than giving advice to others, sharing your own experiences.

We all have to keep learning. I ask patients that use mucuna to collaborate: please send to me your comments by email:

rafael@gonzalezmaldonado.com

Thank you.

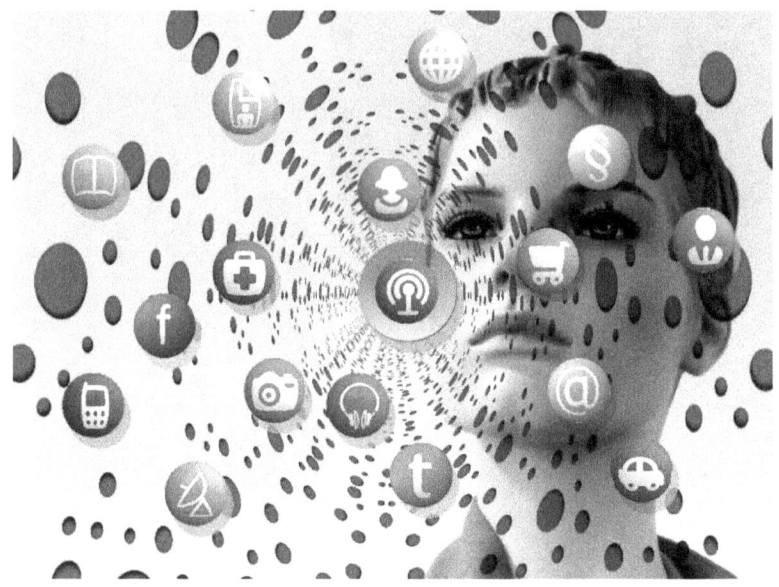

TO BUY MUCUNA AND DO CONSULTATIONS

The offer of mucuna products is wide and information is confusing. Mucuna should never be taken without medical control. These are my links to general or professional consultations:

www.parkinson-mucuna.com
www.levodopa.net
www.neurologo.biz

12. Buy mucuna *online.* Do consultations

I reiterate it. Buy and consume mucuna requires a neurologist and the direct advice of your regular doctor.

Online mucuna is a very profitable business. It is sold as an herbal product with no need for a prescription.

The variety of extracts of mucuna offered is huge, and the consumer may get lost in the plethora of powders, drops, capsules and tablets. For that reason, in Chapter 8, I have summarized the majority of them, and I have given some general guidelines in Chapter 9.

You must verify the source and destination. Customs blocks often products purchased online. In the United States there is no difficulty in getting any kind of product. But currently is difficult to purchase them from Europe.

For now, just a few European businesses, ship mucuna to online buyers. The most well-known are based in France (for example, the French version of Amazon) or Andorra (certain pharmacies).

In Spain, mucuna is sold in some pharmacies (the pioneers are found in Barcelona), and other companies have opened retail outlets.

The law has changed recently. From 2015 on, antiparkinsonian drugs that are not sold in Spain will can be ordered in some pharmacies, if a prescription is provided.

The purchase can be made online but only with pharmacies having a physical location. In the case of these, obviously it will be easier to get mucuna which does not require a prescription.

By now (summer 2014) the main options for those wanting to purchase mucuna in Spain have been described in Chapter 8, including different brands and forms. The following is a summary.

UNITED STATES

In the United States there are no problems for almost any preparation of mucuna including low doses that are sold as dietary supplements and which are ideal for starting treatment.

EUROPE

In France and Andorra I have found mucuna preparations available from 50 to 120 milligrams per capsule. These sources currently send it to Spain without problems.

SPAIN

Ebay is an option for any product, but I advise against it unless you have absolute trust in the provider. The package must be received intact.

Europeans have the option of visiting websites from the United States to obtain information about mucuna and make comparisons, but these sources do not send the product to Spain.

You can get mucuna extracts manufactured in Germany and France, but they are only sent from France or Andorra. In Amazon-France some brands are supplied.

Other online businesses have representatives in Spain (Anastore, Biovea, Carethy) and the product can be purchased in 3-4 days. Mucuna can be obtained in some pharmacies in Barcelona and this will be even easier starting in 2015.

RECOMMENDED LINKS AND CONSULTATIONS

www.levodopa.net
www.parkinson-mucuna.com

Addresses for purchasing mucuna change or expand daily. At my websites www.parkinson-mucuna.com and www.levodopa.net I describe what I consider the most desirable presentations and I compare several suppliers. I must repeat my warning that mucuna should never be taken without medical supervision. On these websites I attempt to maintain up-to-date information.

If you need to consultation specific cases you may also visit my professional website:

www.neurologo.biz

BIBLIOGRAPHY

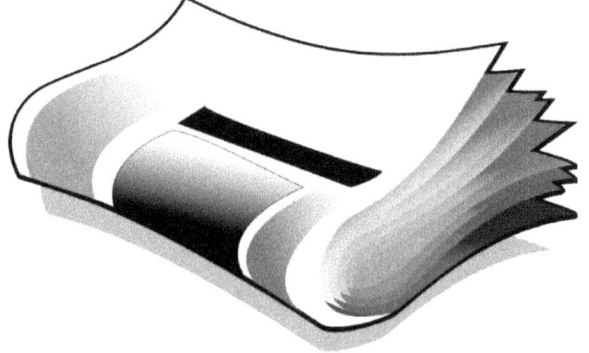

Scientific literature and other references on *mucuna pruriens* I've included throughout this book.

Bibliography

1. **Guggenheim M.** *Dioxyphenylalanine, a new amino acid from Vicia faba.* Z Physiol Chem 1913; 88:276.

2. **Hornykiewicz O.** *A brief history of levodopa.* J Neurol 2010; 257:S249-252.

3. **Hornykiewicz O.** *L-DOPA: from a biologically inactive amino acid to a successful therapeutic agent.* Amino Acids 2002; 23:65-70.

4. **Salat D, Tolosa E.** *Levodopa in the treatment of Parkinson's disease: current status and new developments.* J Parkinsons Dis 2013; 3:255-269.

5. **Soares AR et al.** *The role of L-DOPA in plants.* Plant Signal Behav 2014; 4:9. pii: e28275.

6. **Guidotti BB et al.** *The effects of dopamine on root growth and enzyme activity in soybean seedlings.* Plant Signal Behav 2013; 8.pii: e25477.

7. **Rehr SS, Janzen DH, Feeny PP.** *L-dopa in legume seeds: a chemical barrier to insect attack.* Science 1973; 181:81-82.

8. **Tomita-Yokotani K et al.** *Fate of allelopathic substances in space--allelopathy of velvet bean plant and gravity.* Biol Sci Space 2004; 18:91.

9. **Fujii Y.** *Allelopathy in the natural and agricultural ecosystems and isolation of potent allelochemicals from Velvet bean (Mucuna pruriens) and Hairy vetch (Vicia villosa).* Biol Sci Space 2003; 17:6-13.

10. **Ramya KB, Thaakur S.** *Herbs containing L- Dopa: An update.* Anc Sci Life 2007; 27:50-55.

11. **Spengos M, Vassilopoulos D.** *Improvement of Parkinson's disease after Vicia faba consumption.* Book of Abstracts, Ninth International Symposium on Parkinson's disease. 1988;46.

12. **Rabey JM et al.** *Improvement of parkinsonian features correlate with high plasma levodopa values after broad bean (Vicia faba) consumption.* J Neurol Neurosurg Psychiatry 1992; 55:725-727.

13. **Rabey JM et al.** *Broad bean (Vicia faba) consumption and Parkinson's disease.* Adv Neurol 1993; 60:681-684.

14. **Mehran SM.** *Simultaneous determination of levodopa and carbidopa from fava bean, green peas and*

green beans by high performance liquid gas chromatography. J Clin Diagn Res 2013; 7:1004-1007.

15. **Brod LS, Aldred JL, Nutt JG.** *Are high doses of carbidopa a concern? A randomized, clinical trial in Parkinson's disease.* Mov Disord 2012; 27:750-753.

16. **Durso R et al.** *Variable absorption of carbidopa affects both peripheral and central levodopa metabolism.* J Clin Pharmacol 2000; 40:854-860.

17. **Kempster PA et al.** *Motor effects of broad beans (Vicia faba) in Parkinson's disease: single dose studies.* Asia Pac J Clin Nutr 1993; 2:85-89.

18. **Vered Y et al.** *Bioavailability of levodopa after comsumption of Vicia faba seedlings by Parkinsonian patients and control subjects.* Clin Neuropharmacol 1994; 17:138-146.

19. **Goyoaga C et al.** *Content and distribution of vicine, convicine and L-DOPA during germination and seedling growth of twoVicia faba L. varieties.* Europ Food Research Techn 2008; 227: 1537-1542.

20. **Kirakosyan A et al.** *The production of L-dopa and isoflavones in seeds and seedlings of different cultivars of*

Vivia faba L. (fava bean). Evidence-Based Integrative Medicine 2004; 1:131-135.

21. **Ramírez-Moreno JM, Salguero I, Romaskevych O, Durán, MC.** *Consumo de habas (Vicia faba) y enfermedad de Parkinson: una fuente natural de L-dopa a tener en cuenta.* Carta al editor. Neurología 2013. doi:10.1016/j.nrl.2013.08.006.

22. **Ladha SS, Walker R, Shill, HA.** *Case of neuroleptic malignant-like syndrome precipitated by abrupt fava bean discontinuance.* Mov Disord 2005; 20:630-631.

23. **Apaydin H, Ertan S, Ozekmekçi, S.** *Broad bean (Vicia faba)--a natural source of L-dopa--prolongs "on" periods in patients with Parkinson's disease who have "on-off" fluctuations.* Mov Disord 2000; 15:164-166.

24. **Holden, K.** *Fava Beans, Levodopa, and Parkinson's Disease.* http://www.scienzavegetariana.it/nutrizione/favabeans.html.

25. **Raguthu L, Varanese S, Flancbaum L, Tayler E, Di Rocco A.** *Fava beans and Parkinson's disease: useful 'natural supplement' or useless risk? .* Eur J Neurol. 2009; 16:e171.

26. **Katzenschlager R et al.** *Mucuna pruriens in Parkinson's disease: a double blind clinical and pharmacological study.* J Neurol Neurosurg Psychiatry 2004; 75:1677.

27. **Damodaran M, Ramaswamy R.** *Isolation ol L-dopa from the sedes of Mucuna pruriens.* Biochem J 1937; 31:2149-2451.

28. **Agostini K, Sazima M. Galetto L.** *Nectar production dynamics and sugar composition in two Mucuna species (Leguminosae, Faboideae) with different specialized pollinators.* Naturwissenschaften 2011; 98:933-942.

29. **Brunner B, Beaver J, Flores L.** *Mucuna.* http://prorganico.info/ mucuna.pdf.

30. **Madzimure J et al.** *Performance of Mashona doelings supplemented with different levels of velvet bean (Mucuna pruriens L. DC. var. utilis) seed meal.* Trop Anim Health Prod 2014; 46:901-904.

31. **Vadivel V et al.** *Evaluation of velvet bean meal as an alternative protein ingredient for poultry feed.* Animal 2011; 5:67-73.

32. **Tse GG et al.** *Case of Levodopa Toxicity from Ingestion of Mucuna gigantea.* Hawaii J Med Public Health 2013; 72: 157–160.

33. **Lieu CA et al.** *The Antiparkinsonian and Antidyskinetic Mechanisms of Mucuna pruriens in the MPTP-Treated Nonhuman Primate.* Evid Based Complement Alternat Med 2012; 2012:840247.

34. **Manyam BV, Dhanasekaran M, Hare TA.** *Effect of antiparkinson drug HP-200 (Mucuna pruriens) on the central monoaminergic neurotransmitters.* Phytother Res 2004; 18:97-101.

35. **Manyam BV, Dhanasekaran M, Hare TA.** *Neuroprotective effects of the antiparkinson drug Mucuna pruriens.* Phytother Res 2004; 18:706-712.

36. **Burgess, S, Hemmer, A y Myhrman, R.** *Examination of raw and roasted Mucuna pruriens for tumerogenic substances.* Tropical and Subtropical Agroecosystems 2003; 1:287–293.

37. **Der Giessen RV, Olanow W, Lees A, Wagner H.** *Method for preparing Mucuna pruriens see extract.* United States Patent, US 7,470,441 B2, Dec. 30, 2008.

38. **Kuber R, Thaakur S.** *Herbs containing L-Dopa: an update.* Ancient Science of Life 2007; XXVII:50-55.

39. **Randhir R, Kwon YI, Shetty K.** *Improved health-relevant functionality in dark germinated Mucuna pruriens sprouts by elicitation with peptide and phytochemical elicitors.* Bioresour Technol 2009;100:4507-4514.

40. **Pras N et al.** *Mucuna pruriens: improvement of the biotechnological production of the anti-Parkinson drug L-dopa by plant cell selection.* Pharm World Sci 1993; 15:263-268.

41. **Raghavendra S et al.** *Enhanced production of L-DOPA in cell cultures of Mucuna pruriens L. and Mucuna prurita H.* Nat Prod Res 2012; 26:792-801.

42. **Chattopadhyay S, Datta SK, Mahato SB.** *Production of L-DOPA from cell suspension culture of Mucuna pruriens f. pruriens.* Plant Cell Rep 1994; 13:519-522.

43. **Aguilera Y et al.** *Changes in nonnutritional factors and antioxidant activity during germination of nonconventional legumes.* J Agric Food Chem 2013; 61:8120-8125.

44. **Uma S, Gurumoorthi P.** *Dietary antioxidant activities in different germplasms of Mucuna.* J Med Food 2013; 16:618-24.

45. **Woodson RE et al.** *Rauwolfia: Botany, Pharmacognosy, Chemistry and Pharmacology.* Little Brown & Co, Boston 1957.

46. **Dev S.** *Ancient-modern concordance in Ayurvedic plants: some examples.* Env Health Perspect 1999; 107:783-789.

47. **Alleman RJJr et al.** *A blend of chlorophytum borivilianum and velvet bean increases serum growth hormone in exercise-trained men.* Nutr Metab Insights 2011; 4:55-63.

48. **Obogwu MB, Akindele AJ, Adeyemi OO.** *Hepatoprotective and in vivo antioxidant activities of the hydroethanolic leaf extract of Mucuna pruriens (Fabaceae) in antitubercular drugs and alcohol models.* Chin J Nat Med 2014; 12:273-283.

49. **Majekodunmi SO et al.** *Evaluation of the anti-diabetic properties of Mucuna pruriens seed extract.* Asian Pac J Trop Med 2011; 4:632-636.

50. **Dharmarajan SK y Arumugam KM.** *Comparative evaluation of flavone from Mucuna pruriens and coumarin from Ionidium suffruticosum for hypolipidemic activity in rats fed with high fat diet.* Lipids Health Dis 2012; 11:126.

51. **Pant MC et al.** *Blood sugar and total cholesterol lowering effect of Glycine soja (Sieb and Zucc.), Mucunapruriens (D.C.) and Dolichos biflorus (Linn.) seed diets in normal fasting albino rats.* Indian J Med Res 1968; 56:1808-1012.

52. **Grover, JK, Rathi, SS y Vats, V.** *Amelioration of experimental diabetic neuropathy and gastropathy in rats following oral administration of plant (Eugenia jambolana, Mucuna pruriens and Tinospora cordifolia) extracts.* Indian J Exp Biol 2002; 40:273-276.

53. **Golbabapour S et al.** *Acute toxicity and gastroprotective role of M. pruriens in ethanol-induced gastric mucosal injuries in rats.* Biomed Res Int 2013; 2013: 974185.

54. **Suresh S, Prakash, S.** *Effect of Mucuna pruriens (Linn.) on sexual behavior and sperm parameters in streptozotocin-induced diabetic male rat.* J Sex Med 2012; 9:3066-3078.

55. **Suresh S, Prithiviraj E, Prakash S.** *Dose- and time-dependent effects of ethanolic extract of Mucuna pruriens Linn. seed on sexual behaviour of normal male rats.* J Ethnopharmacol 2009; 122:497-501.

56. **Singh AP et al.** *Mucuna pruriens and its major constituent L-DOPA recover spermatogenic loss by combating ROS, loss of mitochondrial membrane potential and apoptosis.* PLoS One 2013; 8:e54655.

57. **Ahmad MK et al.** *Effect of Mucuna pruriens on semen profile and biochemical parameters in seminal plasma of infertile men.* Fertil Steril 2008; 90:627-635.

58. **Shukla KK et al.** *Mucuna pruriens improves male fertility by its action on the hypothalamus-pituitary-gonadal axis.* Fertil Steril 2009; 92:1934-1940.

59. **Champatisingh D et al.** *Anticataleptic and antiepileptic activity of ethanolic extract of leaves of Mucuna pruriens: A study on role of dopaminergic system in epilepsy in albino rats.* Indian J Pharmacol 2011; 43:197-199.

60. **Scirè A et al.** *The belonging of gpMuc, a glycoprotein from Mucuna pruriens seeds, to the Kunitz-type trypsin inhibitor family explains its direct anti-snake venom activity.* Phytomedicine 2011; 18:887-895.

61. **Hope-Onyekwere NS et al.** *Effects of Mucuna pruriens protease inhibitors on Echis carinatus venom.* Phytother Res 2012; 26:1913-1919.

62. **Fung SY, Tan NH, Sim SM.** *Protective effects of Mucuna pruriens seed extract pretreatment against cardiovascular and respiratory depressant effects of Calloselasma rhodostoma (Mala7yan pit viper) venom in rats.* Trop Biomed 2010; 27:366-372.

63. **Fung SY et al.** *Effect of Mucuna pruriens Seed Extract Pretreatment on the Responses of Spontaneously Beating Rat Atria and Aortic Ring to Naja sputatrix (Javan Spitting Cobra) Venom.* Evid Based Complement Alternat Med 2012; 2012:486390.

64. **Fung SY et al.** *Mucuna pruriens Linn. seed extract pretreatment protects against cardiorespiratory and neuromuscular depressant effects of Naja sputatrix (Javan spitting cobra) venom in rats.* Indian J Exp Biol 2011; 49:254-259.

65. **Manyam BV.** *Paralysis agitans and levodopa in "Ayurveda": ancient Indian medical treatise.* Mov Disord 1990; 5:47-48.

66. **Ovallath S, Deepa P.** *The history of parkinsonism: descriptions in ancient Indian medical literature.* Mov Disord 2013; 28:566-568.

67. **Manyam BV, Sánchez-Ramos JR.** *Traditional and complementary therapies in Parkinson's disease.* Adv Neurol 1999; 80:565-574.

68. **Nagashayana N et al.** *Association of L-DOPA with recovery following Ayurveda medication in Parkinson's disease.* J Neurol Sci 2000; 176:124-127.

69. **González Maldonado R.** *Tratamientos heterodoxos en la enfermedad de Parkinson, 2013.* Amazon.es.

70. **Misra L, Wagner H.** *Extraction of bioactive principles from Mucuna pruriens seeds.* Indian J Biochem Biophys 2007; 44:56-60.

71. **Vaidya AB et al.** *Treatment of Parkinson's disease with the cowhage plant-Mucuna pruriens Bak.* Neurol India 1978; 26:171-176.

72. **González Maldonado R.** *El extraño caso del Dr. Parkinson.* Grupo Editorial Universitario. Granada, 1997. : s.n.

73. **Parkinson's Disease Study Group, PDSG.** *An alternative medicine treatment for Parkinson's disease:*

results of a multicenter clinical trial. HP-200 in PD Study Group. J Altern Complement Med 1995; 1:249-255.

74. **Manyam BV.** *Beans (Mucuna pruriens) for Parkinson's disease: an herbal alternative.* www.parkinson.org/beans.htem (2003).

75. **Suchowersky O et al.** *Practice Parameter: Neuroprotective strategies and alternative therapies for Parkinson disease (an evidence-based review). Report of the Quality Standards Subcommittee of the American Academy of Neurology.* Neurology 2006; 66:976-972.

76. **Hussian G, Manyam BV.** *Mucuna pruriens proves more effective than L-DOPA in Parkinson's disease animal model.* Phytotherapy Research 1997; 11:419–423.

77. **Behari M et al.** *Experiences of Parkinson's disease in India.* Lancet Neurol 2002; 1:258-262.

78. **Lieu CA et al.** *A water extract of Mucuna pruriens provides long-term amelioration of parkinsonism with reduced risk for dyskinesias.* Parkinsonism Relat Disord 2010; 16:458-465.

79. **Pathan AA et al.** *Mucuna pruriens attenuates haloperidol-induced orofacial dyskinesia in rats.* Nat Prod Res 2011; 25:764-771.

80. **Lampariello LR et al.** *The Magic Velvet Bean of Mucuna pruriens.* J Tradit Complement Med 2012; 2:331-339.

81. **Kasture S et al.** *Assessment of symptomatic and neuroprotective efficacy of Mucuna pruriens seed extract in rodent model of Parkinson's disease.* Neurotox Res 2009; 15:111-122.

82. **Yadav SK et al.** *Comparison of the neuroprotective potential of Mucuna pruriens seed extract with estrogen in 1-methyl-4-phenyl-1,2,3,6-tetrahydropyridine (MPTP)-induced PD mice model.* Neurochem Int 2014; 65:1-13.

83. **Dhanasekaran M, Tharakan B, Manyam BV.** *Antiparkinson drug--Mucuna pruriens shows antioxidant and metal chelating activity.* Phytother Res 2008; 22:6-11.

84. **Tharakan B et al.** *Anti-Parkinson botanical Mucuna pruriens prevents levodopa induced plasmid and genomic DNA damage.* Phytother Res 2007; 21:1124-1126.

85. **Yadav SK et al.** *Mucuna pruriens seed extract reduces oxidative stress in nigrostriatal tissue and improves neurobehavioral activity in paraquat-induced Parkinsonian mouse model.* Neurochem Int 2013; 62:1039-1047.

86. **Lees A, Olanow WC, Der Giessen RV, Wagner H.** *Mucuna pruriens and extracts thereof for the treatment of neurological diseases.* Patent WO 2004039385-A2, 2004, May 13.

87. **Mahajani SS et al.** *Bioavailability of L-DOPA from HP-200 : a formulation of seed powder of Mucuna pruriens (Bak) : a pharmacokinetic and pharmacodynamic study.* Phytotherapy Research 1996; 10:254-256.

88. **Pruthi SC, Pruthy P.** *Ayurvedic composition for the treatment of disorders of the nervous system including Parkinson's disease.* Patent US 6106839 A. https://www.google.com/patents/US6106839.

89. **Manyam BV, Dhanasekaran M, Cassady JM.** *Anti-Parkinson's disease pharmaceutical and method of use.* United States Patent 20050202111-A1. http://www.freepatentsonline.com/y2005/0202111.html.

90. **González Maldonado R.** *Parkinson y estrés.* CreateSpace 2013, Amazon.

91. **González Maldonado R.** *Conjeturas de un neurólogo que escuchó a mil parkinsonianos.* CreateSpace 2014, Amazon.

92. **Munhoz RP, Teive HA.** *Darkening of white hair in Parkinson's disease during use of levodopa rich Mucuna pruriens extract powder.* Arq Neuropsiquiatr 2013; 71:133.

93. **Infante ME et al.** *Outbreak of acute toxic psychosis attributed to Mucuna pruriens.* Lancet 1990; 336:1129.

94. **Bertoldi M, Gonsalvi M, Voltattorni CB.** *Green tea polyphenols: novel irreversible inhibitors of dopa decarboxylase.* Biochem Biophys Res Commun 2001; 284:90-93.

95. **Kang KS et al.** *Dual beneficial effects of (-) epigallocatechin-3-gallate on levodopa methylation and hippocampal neurodegeneration: in vitro and in vivo studies.* PLoS One 2010; 5(8):e11951. doi: 10.1371/journal.

96. **Guo S et al.** *Protective effects of green tea polyphenols in the 6-OHDA rat model of Parkinson's disease through inhibition of ROS-NO pathway.* Biol Psychiatry 2007; 62:1353-1362.

97. **Hinz M, Stein A, Uncini T.** *Relative nutritional deficiencies associated with centrally acting monoamines.* Int J Gen Med 2012; 5:413-430.

98. **Hinz M, Stein A, Uncini T.** *Amino acid management of Parkinson's disease: a case study.* Int J Gen Med 2011; 4:165-174.

99. **Kim TH et al.** *Herbal Medicines for Parkinson's Disease: A Systematic Review of Randomized Controlled Trials.* PLoS ONE 2012; 7: e35695. doi:10.1371.

100. **Lyytinen J et al.** *Entacapone and selegiline with L-dopa in patients with Parkinson's disease: an interaction study.* Parkinsonism Relat Disord 2000; 6:215-222.

101. **Cassani E et al.** *Natural therapy: Mucuna pruriens. A possible alternative in developing countries.* 18th Movement Disorders Society Meeting, Stockholm, june 2014.

102. **Cassani E et al.** *Mucuna pruriens: A new strategy for Parkinson's disease treatment in Africa. An update.* 18th Movement Disorders Society Meeting, Stockholm, june 2014.

TABLE OF CONTENTS

Index 7

Introduction 9

    LEVODOPA IS CONVERTED TO DOPAMINE 13

    PARKINSON'S PATIENTS LACK OF DOPAMINE 13

    DOPAMINE INCREASED AFTER TAKING LEVODOPA 14

    BEGINNING TO WALK, THEY BEGAN TO VOMIT 14

    SINEMET AND MADOPAR PREVENT VOMITING 15

    PATIENTS TREATED WITH SYNTHETIC LEVODOPA 16

    FOUR TYPES OF SINEMET 16

    LEVODOPA + BENSERAZIDE (MADOPAR) 17

    "STABILIZED" LEVODOPA (STALEVO) 17

    LEVODOPA AS A DEFENSE AGAINST ITS NEIGHBORS 18

    OTHER PLANTS CONTAINING LEVODOPA 19

2.   Beans contain levodopa 21

    CONSUMING BEANS IMPROVES PARKINSON'S 21

    A SERVING OF BEANS IS HALF A SINEMET 21

    JUST A LITTLE LEVODOPA WORKS 22

LEVODOPA PLUS CARBIDOPA IS MORE EFECTIVE 23

BEANS ENRICHED WITH CARBIDOPA 24

POWDERED DRY BEANS HAVE LITTLE LEVODOPA 25

SEEDBED TO COLLECT BEAN SPROUTS 26

DOSAGE MUST BE ADAPTED TO EACH CASE 27

BEANS ARE MORE EFFECTIVE IN PATIENTS 27

NEUROLEPTIC SYNDROME AFTER CESSATION OF BEANS 28

BEANS REDUCE "ON-OFF" FLUCTUATIONS 28

SEARCHING FOR PLANTS WITH MORE LEVODOPA 29

3. Mucuna, a bean that grows in the tropics 31

FURRY BEAN GROWING IN THE TROPICS 31

A SHRUB AS A VINE 32

ITS FLOWERS ARE POLLINATED BY BATS 32

PODS AND SEEDS 33

NAMED "PRURIENS" BECAUSE OF THE ITCH 33

FOOD, FORAGE OR GREEN MANURE 34

AN ANCIENT MEDICINE 35

TOXICITY OF MUCUNA AND OTHERS LEGUMES 35

LEVODOPA AND MORE 36

50 KNOWN INGREDIENTS, OTHERS REMAIN 36

- OTHER PLANTS THAT CONTAIN LEVODOPA 37
- MUCUNA CONTAINS MORE LEVODOPA 38
- MUCUNA CAN PROVIDE OTHER BENEFITS 39

4. From the herbalist shop to the pharmacy 41
   - HERBS THAT HEAL 42
   - MUCUNA AS PANACEA 42
   - GROWTH HORMONE BOOSTER 43
   - LOWERING OF CHOLESTEROL AND GLUCOSE................................ 43
   - AN APHRODISIAC THAT IMPROVES SEMEN 44
   - IT ACTS AGAINST EPILEPSY AND AGAINST CATALEPSY............... 44
   - SNAKE POISON ANTIDOTE 45
   - IMPROVES BOWEL MOVEMENT 45
   - KAMPAVATA IS PARKINSON'S DISEASE 46
   - ITS NAME WAS ATMAGUPTA... 46
   - AYURVEDA IN TREATING PARKINSON 47
   - THE SEEDS ARE COOKED IN COW'S MILK 47
   - HIDDEN INGREDIENTS IN MUCUNA 48

5. Mucuna works better than Sinemet 51
   - FIRST DESCRIPTIONS 51
   - MUCUNA SEED POWDER 52

ZANDOPA: A MEDICINE WITH MUCUNA 53

IMPROVEMENT IN MICE DOUBLES OR TRIPLES 53

ENDORSED BY THE AMERICAN ACADEMY 54

"CITIUS, ALTIUS, FORTIUS ET DURABILIUS" 56

TWICE AS EFFECTIVE 56

THE PROBLEM OF VOLUME 57

MUCUNA WITH CARBIDOPA 58

MUCUNA DOES NOT PRODUCE DYSKINESIA 60

LONG-TERM MUCUNA WITHOUT DYSKINESIA 60

MUCUNA IMPROVES HALOPERIDOL-INDUCED DYSKINESIA 61

MUCUNA IS NEUROPROTECTIVE 62

CHELATING AND ANTIOXIDANT PROPERTIES 63

MUCUNA IMPROVES BRAIN FUNCTION IN RATS 63

DOSAGE DOES NOT INCREASE OVER TIME! 64

6. Extracts of mucuna patented by neurologists 67

DR. OLANOW AND DR. LEES 68

PATENTS OF EXTRACTS OF MUCUNA 70

ZANDOPA AND A COCKTAIL WITH MUCUNA 70

AN EXTRA-CONCENTRATED EXTRACT 71

MORE BENEFITS THAN CONVENTIONAL LEVODOPA 72

A WIDE THERAPEUTIC WINDOW 72

PATIENTS GET BETTER SOONER WITH MUCUNA 73

THE DURABLE EFFECT OF MUCUNA 73

LESS TOXIC THAN SYNTHETIC LEVODOPA 73

COMBINATION THERAPY MAY BE DELAYED 74

MUCUNA FOR ALMOST EVERYTHING.. 74

HIDDEN INGREDIENTS IN MUCUNA 75

GRAY HAIR REVERSAL USING MUCUNA 76

MUCUNA IS MORE THAN LEVODOPA... 77

7. Contraindications and warnings... 79

PATIENTS DO NOT KNOW WHAT THEY ARE TAKING 79

THEY DESPISE WHAT THEY DO NOT KNOW................................... 80

WHY ARE THERE NO FREQUENT MAJOR PROBLEMS? 81

CONTRAINDICATIONS OF LEVODOPA... 82

DRUGS THAT INTERACT WITH LEVODOPA...................................... 83

SIDE EFFECTS WITH LEVODOPA 84

SPECIFIC WARNING ABOUT MUCUNA... 85

BE CAREFUL WHEN COMBINING MUCUNA AND GREEN TEA........ 86

8. Dosage and presentations 89

BEFORE USING MUCUNA 89

	A STRATEGY TO START USING MUCUNA	90
	CAREFUL WITH MISTAKES IN DOSAGE	91
	BE CAREFUL WHEN BUYING MUCUNA	92
	PRICE SHOULD NOT MATTER AT THE BEGINNING	92
	PRESENTATIONS	93
a)	Mucuna powder	95
	ZANDOPA HP-200.	95
	COMMON MISTAKES IN PRESCRIBING ZANDOPA	96
b)	Mucuna in very low doses (15-30 mg)	98
	HIMALAYA	98
	ADVANCE PHYSICIAN	98
c)	Mucuna in low doses (50-60 mg)	99
	SOLARAY DOPA-BEAN	99
	AYURVANA MUCUNA	99
	BONUSAN	99
d)	Mucuna in medium doses (75-100 mg)	100
	VITAWORLD	100
	ANASTORE	100
	BIOVEA MUCUNA DOPA	101
e)	Mucuna in high doses (more than 100 mg)	101

	NOW DOPA MUCUNA	101
f)	Tincture or Mucuna drops	102
g)	Mucuna mixed with other substances	102

9. Testimonials from those who take mucuna 105

    FORUMS ON MUCUNA 105

    CONCLUSIONS DERIVED FROM THESE FORUMS 106

10. How to start taking mucuna: case studies 109

    MUCUNA IS NOT FOR EVERYONE 109

    AN INCREASE IN MUCUNA MEANS A DECREASE IN PHARMACEUTICAL DRUGS 110

    NOT FOR PEOPLE WITHOUT PARKINSON'S DISEASE 110

    PARKINSON'S DIAGNOSIS UP TO 55 YEARS 111

    PARKINSON'S DIAGNOSIS AT 75 YEARS-OLD 112

    TRIALS WITH SINEMET-FREE PATIENTS 113

    PATIENTS TAKING LOW DOSES OF SINEMET 114

    PATIENTS TAKING A MEDIUM DOSE OF SINEMET 115

    PATIENTS TAKING STALEVO 117

    TAKING RASAGILINE PLUS SINEMET 118

    PATIENTS WHO ONLY TAKE RASAGILINE 119

    PATIENTS TAKING ONLY DOPAMINE AGONISTS 121

PATIENTS WHO TAKE AMANTADINE	122
PATIENTS TAKING STALEVO AND RASAGILINE	123
PATIENTS WHO TRIED APOMORPHINE	124
POLYPHARMACY AND MANY YEARS OF PARKINSON'S	124
WHEN PATIENTS TAKE OTHER DRUGS	125
MUCUNA ONLY AS THE "RESCUE" DOSE	125
ADDING CARBIDOPA TO MUCUNA	126
11. The future of mucuna	**129**
CARBIDOPA AND AMINO ACIDS	130
MUCUNA: THE LEVODOPA FOR THE POOR	131
NEUROLOGISTS IN GHANA AND ZAMBIA	132
IT IS RIGHT TO STUDY THIS OPTION	133
WHY IS IT SO EXPENSIVE IN THE WEST?	133
WHY IS MUCUNA NOT PRESCRIBED BY NEUROLOGISTS?	134
MUCUNA AND OTHER PLANTS	135
CHEMISTRY PROFESSOR PREPARES HIS MUCUNA	135
PATIENTS CAN HELP A LOT	137
12. Buy mucuna *online*. Do consultations	**141**
UNITED STATES	142
EUROPE	143

SPAIN	143
RECOMMENDED LINKS AND CONSULTATIONS	144
Bibliography	147
TABLE OF CONTENTS	165

FINIS

www.ingramcontent.com/pod-product-compliance
Lightning Source LLC
Chambersburg PA
CBHW051518170526
45165CB00002B/513